Epilepsy in Our View

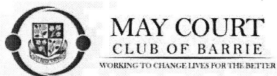

Comments on *Epilepsy in Our View: Stories from Friends and Families of People Living with Epilepsy*

It sure would have been helpful for my wife and children to have read *Epilepsy in Our View* when they were first faced with the knowledge that their husband and father had a seizure disorder.

A reader

I would recommend that all patients with epilepsy own a copy of this book. It should also be included in medical bookstores and medical and community libraries.

Tonya F. Fuller, Doody's Health Sciences Book Review Journal

Comments on *Epilepsy in Our Experience: Accounts of Health Care Professionals*

I felt very reassured knowing that other health care professionals have faced similar situations and am thankful for their willingness to share them.

A reader

This latest edition to the Brainstorms series undoubtedly will have many readers. All of them will be grateful to the editor and the fourscore contributors for the production of this unusual book.

Harry Meinardi, Epilepsia

Comments on *Epilepsy in Our Lives: Women Living with Epilepsy*

As a woman with epilepsy I will keep it with me for the support I need when next I encounter "the world that doesn't understand me."

A reader

I read *Epilepsy in Our Lives* and just wish books like this had been published when I was a kid growing up with epilepsy. It was wonderful to read about what others with epilepsy were experiencing that I could relate to.

A reader

Comments on *Epilepsy in Our Words:*
Personal Accounts of Living with Seizures

You cannot imagine how much *Epilepsy in Our Words* has helped me to accept epilepsy as something I'm just going to have to live with. Just knowing that I'm not the only one that has gone through some of these experiences makes it easier.

A reader

. . . the first book of its kind.

USA Today

Comments on *Epilepsy in Our World:*
Stories of Living with Seizures from Around the World

This book is really wonderful! . . . Please receive all my congratulations for these books, for your continued project, your continuous learning and education how to understand, help, and treat people with epilepsy.

A reader

Comments on *Epilepsy on Our Terms:*
Stories by Children with Seizures and Their Parents

Thank you so much for your latest Brainstorms book. I have just finished reading it and I must tell you that I felt every emotion imaginable. Some of those children seemed to have a better grasp of their situation than I have. I cried, I laughed, and experienced all the feelings in between. The parents' stories were truly heartbreaking. To watch your child go through everything that epilepsy brings with it must be a horrifying thing. Most told their stories in such a realistic way that I had a mental image of just what they were going through.

A reader

To my knowledge, this is the first time families express themselves in detail and can express how the disorder is perceived "from the inside." Such an approach should prove most useful for the newly affected families who are suddenly faced with a disorder they had never heard of and who discover that their child has this mysterious disease.

Olivier Dulac, *Epilepsia*

Other Brainstorms books

Epilepsy in Our Experience:
Accounts of Health Care Professionals

Epilepsy in Our Lives:
Women Living with Epilepsy

Epilepsy in Our Words:
Personal Accounts of Living with Seizures

Epilepsy in Our World:
Stories of Living with Seizures from Around the World

Epilepsy on Our Terms:
Stories by Children with Seizures and Their Parents

Epilepsy in Our View

Stories from Friends and Families of People Living with Epilepsy

Steven C. Schachter, MD

Director of Research
Department of Neurology
Beth Israel Deaconess Medical Center

and

Professor of Neurology
Harvard Medical School
Boston, Massachusetts

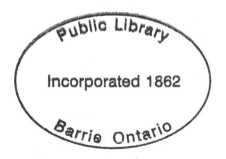

OXFORD
UNIVERSITY PRESS

2008

OXFORD
UNIVERSITY PRESS

Oxford University Press, Inc., publishes works that further
Oxford University's objective of excellence
in research, scholarship, and education.

Oxford   New York
Auckland   Cape Town   Dar es Salaam   Hong Kong   Karachi
Kuala Lumpur   Madrid   Melbourne   Mexico City   Nairobi
New Delhi   Shanghai   Taipei   Toronto

With offices in
Argentina   Austria   Brazil   Chile   Czech Republic   France   Greece
Guatemala   Hungary   Italy   Japan   Poland   Portugal   Singapore
South Korea   Switzerland   Thailand   Turkey   Ukraine   Vietnam

Published by Oxford University Press, Inc.
198 Madison Avenue, New York, New York 10016
www.oup.com

Oxford is a registered trademark of Oxford University Press

Library of Congress Cataloging-in-Publication Data
Schachter, Steven C.
Epilepsy in our view : stories from friends and families of people
living with epilepsy / Steven C. Schachter.
   p.   cm.—(Brainstorms)
Includes bibliographical references and index.
ISBN 978-0-19-533087-8
   1. Epileptics—Family relationships.
      2. Epileptics—Biography.
[DNLM: 1. Epilepsy—Personal Narratives.
   2. Family Relations—Personal Narratives.
        WL 385 S291e 2008]
               I. Title.
         II. Brainstorms series.
        RC372.S27   2008
   362.196'85300922—dc22
         2007017457

Cover Art: Volker Rodermund
Faces in a Circle, 2003
On display at the Epilepsy Center Bethel in Bielefeld, Germany
Used with the kind permission of Mrs. Margarete Pfafflins

Printed in the United States of America
on acid-free paper

To my teachers and mentors, especially Lindley Hall, Irving Lewis, and Marcia Wile, for their guidance and encouragement

Contents

Foreword

In the last quarter century we have made great strides in our understanding and treatment of the various forms of epilepsy. Yet seizures continue to be a frightening experience, particularly when they are first witnessed and before their nature is well understood by the person with seizures and the family. The process of adaptation begins with a thorough study of the problem, followed by detailed and patient explanations to all concerned by the medical team. It is particularly important to let the person who experiences seizures, as well as family members, express the feelings and thoughts aroused by these intrusive attacks. Seeing a seizure will always make the adrenaline flow, not only in family members but also in doctors and nurses who witness them, even though they may have seen countless seizures before. The importance of the process of clarification and interpretation, leading finally to acceptance of the condition, must not be minimized. Through this process, emotional reactions to the attacks can be reduced.

While video EEG monitoring of seizures and the recording of the electrical discharges has contributed much to our understanding of the different types of epilepsy and to localization of seizures, it has, on the other hand, removed some of the emphasis on seizure observation and description by family members. One may argue, with some justification, that the emotional state of family members and other witnesses interferes with the accuracy of the descriptions the doctors find so helpful. We have all spoken to parents who cannot clearly recall to which side their child turns during a seizure and what part of the body is most affected. Nevertheless, the observations and descriptions by friends and family members of seizures witnessed in a familiar environment continue to provide valuable clues to the site of onset and types of seizures. The reports in this book teach us a lot about the circumstances surrounding the occurrence of seizures and their medical, social, and emotional impact, and they help us determine the types of medical, psychological, and social intervention required.

Dr. Schachter has perceptively recognized the need to highlight this important aspect of epilepsy by sympathetically listening to the concerns of family members and encouraging them to write about their observations, emotions, innermost thoughts, and worries. The result is a volume of both medical and social importance. The descriptions of seizures and their impact are moving and revealing. They touch on every aspect of life: love, devotion, hope, education, work, driving—but also fear and guilt.

This small book will greatly benefit persons with epilepsy and their families by allowing them to share the experiences of others and by stressing the commonality of their experiences. It is strongly recommended as well to physicians and other healthcare professionals who are involved in the care of persons with epilepsy: it will remind them that the impact of seizures extends to everyone who comes in contact with them and will prepare them for a broader and more effective approach. For this, all of us—patients, families, and workers in epilepsy alike—owe Dr. Schachter a debt of gratitude.

Frederick Andermann, MD, FRCP (C)
Professor of Neurology & Pediatrics
McGill University
Montreal, Quebec, Canada

Foreword

This book is a riveting anthology of reactions to seizures and persons with seizures by those closest to them. There are at least five important lessons to be learned from the text.

First, persons who find themselves relating to someone with epilepsy for the first time will learn what to expect. Although there may be differences in seizure patterns from one person to the next, those who work, interact, or live with a person with a seizure disorder can become more comfortable themselves by reading this book, and more helpful to the person undergoing a seizure.

I wished I had been able to read *Epilepsy in Our Words: Personal Accounts of Living with Seizures* when I first started to have seizures. Just knowing about the experiences of others would have given me some idea of what to expect and I wouldn't have been so terrified at the onset of a seizure or so depressed at the conclusion of one. The same holds true for this book. I wish I had been able to get a copy for my wife and children when I first started to have seizures. Perhaps reading about the experiences of others would have given them some idea of what to expect as well.

Second, we learn of the enormous negative impact that seizure disorders may have on those around us—the fear, pity, guilt, anger, and feelings of helplessness and sometimes hopelessness—generated by epilepsy. These feelings not only are usually unfounded and have the potential of pushing away the person with epilepsy, but also often add to the burden the patient carries. It is said so well by one of the contributors, "In the end, the . . . weight of all the guilt you try to lay on yourself or on others in the family . . . is felt most by the one that has been diagnosed with epilepsy."

Third, the book answers the most common questions asked by a person witnessing a seizure: "What can I do?" The seven-year-old son holds his daddy's hand. The sister remains calm, rubs her sister's back, and is there when the seizure is over. Others are present to offer their reassurance when the seizure is over. "We held her hands and let her sit up and talked to her. This made her less scared." Remaining calm, offering reassurance, and making physical contact are three major themes running through the stories about how to help the person going through a seizure.

Fourth, the text explains to those who experience seizures how they can be helpful to those around them and, in the long run, improve their own situations. Contributors advise persons with epilepsy to let people know what to anticipate and how they can be useful. "She told me what to expect and how to help. Initially I was terrified, feeling an awesome responsibility for her safety . . . As we have gone out together over the past few years, I have become less apprehensive and more confident that I can be helpful if a seizure occurs."

Fifth, the book describes persons with epilepsy who live normal lives in spite of their seizure disorders and the frequently encountered attitude of others that people with epilepsy are different. The book successfully shows that persons with epilepsy cannot be stereotyped and that a person's seizures can range from controlled to very mild and occasional to more frequent and more severe. Thankfully, the majority of persons with epilepsy have good, if not complete, control of their seizures with medication or other therapies. However, whether completely controlled or not, epilepsy has historically been a feared disability, and persons with this diagnosis have been discriminated against, particularly in employment. It is hoped that the Brainstorms books of Dr. Schachter will assist in eradicating some of that discrimination by educating others (including employers) about epilepsy, so that the fear and mystique are dispelled. If not, persons with seizure disorders will have to rely on the antidiscrimination protection afforded by such laws as the Americans with Disabilities Act of 1990.

I want to thank Dr. Schachter for the special interest he has shown in communicating to patients, their families, and friends in a way that contributes to their adjustment to and understanding of epilepsy.

Clayton Boyd
Former Chief of Policy and Program Development
US Department of Veteran Affairs
Vocational Rehabilitation Service
Washington, D.C.

Preface

Epilepsy in Our Words: Personal Accounts of Living with Seizures was compiled in response to requests from people with epilepsy for a book that describes seizures in a readily understandable way. In that book, numerous people with epilepsy describe what they experience before, during, and after seizures, and what life is like with epilepsy.

Dr. Orrin Devinsky and others suggested I put together another book that gives the perspectives of family members and friends of persons with seizures, since epilepsy affects them as well. Therefore, I asked patients of mine to invite their families and friends to write down what they feel and observe when they see a seizure happening. The result of their efforts is this book, which contains descriptions of seizures in the words of mothers, fathers, brothers, sisters, children, friends, colleagues, students, and teachers of people with epilepsy. Many of these people have lived with someone affected by epilepsy for years, and their poignant, candid words reveal a wide range of emotions from frustration and anguish to acceptance and optimism.

The passages in this book illustrate that the first witnessed seizure is often the most vividly remembered. Indeed, the detail found in some of these descriptions is remarkable. These observations are very important to doctors and other health care providers, who must often rely on such descriptions to help establish the diagnosis of epilepsy and to select appropriate therapy. The reader will see that different people may watch the same person having the same type of seizure and yet describe the seizure in different ways.

This book is intended for the families and friends of people with epilepsy, in addition to those with epilepsy themselves. I hope that it will help readers feel connected to a community of people who are struggling with many similar issues and that it will enable readers to gain perspective on their own individual situations and to acquire the words to help express their feelings and observations. In short, this book can serve as a support group in print.

The first section is an introduction to epilepsy and different types of seizures from a medical viewpoint. The second section consists of seizure descriptions, each one written by a different person. Seizure descriptions are numbered. If there is more than one family member or friend describing the same person with epilepsy, then the passage is identified by both a number and a letter. At the beginning of each passage, the relationship of the writer to the person with seizures is given. For example, if "mother" is found at the beginning of a description, the contributor is the mother of the person with seizures. There may also be a number at the end of a passage. This number refers to the seizure description number in *Epilepsy in Our Words: Personal Accounts of Living with Seizures*. For example, if "10" appears at the end of a passage, the seizure description is about the same person who described his or her own seizures in *Epilepsy in Our Words: Personal Accounts of Living with Seizures* under the number "10."

The third section is a collection of statements by some of my patients about living with epilepsy. The fourth section offers suggestions on living safely with epilepsy, a topic raised by a number of contributors to this book, who said that they could respond more effectively to a person having a seizure if they were already familiar with first aid procedures. I encourage people with seizures to share this information with others.

The purpose of this book is to present information and perspectives about seizures and living with epilepsy through the words of actual family members and friends of people with epilepsy in language that is readily understood. Clinical descriptions of seizures and specific recommendations about diagnostic tests, treatment, support services, and driving are important topics but beyond the scope of this book. I strongly encourage people to discuss these topics with their physician and to visit credible websites such as www. epilepsy.com and www.epilepsyfoundation.org.

I invite anyone who would like to share his or her own reactions to this book to write to me at Beth Israel Deaconess Medical Center, Room KS-457, 330 Brookline Avenue, Boston, Massachusetts 02215.

Steven C. Schachter
March 31, 2007

Acknowledgments

The people whose experiences and feelings are recorded in this book have my admiration and gratitude for their courage and frankness. I would like to thank Frederick Andermann for his support of the *Brainstorms* books and for writing a foreword to this book. I am appreciative that Clayton Boyd, a person with epilepsy who dealt with public health policy on epilepsy, also wrote a foreword for the book. I am grateful to Patricia Osborne Shafer and Nancy Santilli for writing the section on living safely with epilepsy. My special thanks go to Cecile Davis, whose hard work and diligence made this project possible. Finally, I wish to acknowledge the enthusiastic support of Cynthia Joyce and Craig Panner.

Introduction

An Overview of Epilepsy and Seizures

A seizure is usually defined as a sudden alteration of behavior due to a temporary change in the electrical functioning of the brain, in particular the outer layer of the brain called the *cortex*. Approximately 1 percent of the population has recurrent seizures. When a person has recurrent seizures over a period of time, he or she is usually diagnosed with epilepsy. Seizures are the main symptoms of epilepsy and the main target for treatment. Seizures can take many different forms, as the descriptions in this book indicate. Usually, any single person experiences only one or two types of seizures, but seizures affect different people in different ways, as this book illustrates.

Sometimes, people with epilepsy can have their seizures triggered, or brought on, by certain identifiable factors. These can include alcohol, strong emotions, intense exercise, flashing lights or loud music, illness and fever, the menstrual period, lack of sleep, and stress. Sometimes there is no identifiable or consistent seizure trigger. Occasionally the trigger is apparent to an onlooker but forgotten by the person having the seizure.

Seizures have a beginning, a middle, and an end. If a person is aware of the beginning, they are said to have a *warning* or *aura*. Auras are actually seizures that affect only a very small part of the brain; enough to cause symptoms but not enough to disrupt consciousness. Doctors may call auras by the term "simple partial seizures"— "simple" means that consciousness is not impaired, and "partial" means that only part of the brain is electrically disrupted by the seizure, while the rest of the brain functions normally.

On the other hand, some people are not aware of the beginning of their seizures and therefore have no warning. This usually means that when the seizure begins, the normal activity of the part of the brain that controls memory is electrically disrupted. This type of seizure is called either an "absence seizure" or a "complex partial seizure"—"complex" refers to the loss of consciousness and reduced awareness of one's surroundings. During a complex partial seizure, the person cannot meaningfully interact with others, and afterwards the person will have no memory of anything that took place during the seizure, even though they may have looked awake. For some people, the seizure begins as a convulsion without any warning.

The middle of the seizure may take several different forms. For those people who have warnings, the aura may simply continue or it may turn into a complex partial seizure or a convulsion. For those who do not have a warning, the seizure may continue as a complex partial seizure or it may evolve into a convulsion. When a convulsion follows a simple partial seizure or a complex partial seizure it is called a "secondarily generalized seizure"—"generalized" means that the electrical disruptions are thought to spread to the entire brain surface. Consequently, all normal functions of the cortex are temporarily shut down.

The end to a seizure represents a transition from the seizure back to a normal state. This period is referred to as the "post-ictal period" (ictus is another name for seizure) and may last from seconds to hours, depending on several factors including which part(s) of the brain were affected by the seizure and whether the person was on anti-seizure medication. If a person had a complex partial seizure or a convulsion, their level of awareness gradually improves during the post-ictal period, much like a person waking up from anesthesia after an operation.

Epilepsy has often been called a hidden disability. In between seizures, most people with epilepsy appear and function normally. Yet no matter how frequently or infrequently a person has seizures, their day-to-day life is often dramatically affected by many factors, including the fear of having a seizure without warning, the possible shame and embarrassment of having a seizure in public, the consequences for employment as well as driving and insurance, and the stigma of epilepsy, which is still prevalent in our culture. As the reader will see, the social consequences of epilepsy are apparent to family members and friends as well, and felt deeply by them.

Seizure Descriptions

Husband My initial introduction to my wife's seizure disorder occurred months before we began dating. We were working in the same office complex when she came into my office one afternoon and sat in the chair across from me. I immediately discerned that something was amiss as she appeared disoriented and did not make much sense when she spoke to me. After a short time, she got up and went into the adjoining office. I immediately followed and stood beside her trying to stop her from wandering around and to ascertain her problem. I now know that she was beginning to "return" as she then started to respond to my questions. She eventually offered an explanation concerning her behavior upon which I asked about medication and whether she had recently taken any. I talked her into taking some and a short while later she was responding normally. It was later that I learned that there was no cause and effect in having her take some medication and her return to normal conduct.

After we started dating, I eventually learned about her seizures, how they manifested themselves and what I should do until she "came back." Since I am a diabetic and have had insulin reactions, understanding her seizures is not a foreign concept to me. Our relationship is not affected at all. My outlook for her medical condition is the same as for my own . . . "C'est la vie!" We watch out for and take care of each other.

The most difficult part of my wife's epilepsy is her lack of memory, both future and past. She lives primarily in the present. We do not have any real "remember when" associations. Many things have been enjoyed and we have traveled around the country but to simply sit and reminisce is not possible as she has very little recall. In this respect, I am alone and wonder what she will remember about our life together should I go first. She also forgets upcoming plans and discussions. Apart from a major item like a vacation she will forget schedules and appointments. I can mention an approaching event and a short while later she will ask if I have any plans for the day or weekend in question. Serious discussions take place and after a short period, it is as if nothing had ever been said.

Everyday life is not disadvantageous. We watch each other for potential medical problems and enjoy life as it comes each day. When her seizures occur they do not last very long and when it is over, the same lovable person is still here. *23*

2

Mother My daughter averages three seizures daily. Usually, she seems to gulp at the onset of a seizure and then falls to the floor. She shakes and is extremely rigid. She will grab at anything or anyone nearby. She often cannot hear or speak, sometimes for as much as twenty minutes, although she is not rigid at this time. Her seizures come without any warning and at all different times of the day (or night). After the seizure has passed, she has no memory of anything that has gone on, and often times does not believe anything has happened.

I am the one who sees all of my daughter's seizures as we are alone a great deal of the day. *58*

3a

Friend The seizures occurred at soccer camp at 19:21 on a Wednesday. The weather was in the 90s and extremely humid.

My friend was laying across a lower bunk-bed with his back in contact with the bed, legs dangling, and his head supported by his peers. He exhibited signs of localized activity of various natures; facial spasms of soft tissue of the maxilla and eyelids; isolated upper extremity tremors. The immediate thought process seemed to be impaired and/or blocked for hours.

3b

Mother Contrary to his usual behavior, my six-month-old little boy was not smiling and was quite nervous. He was touching his ears, scratching himself and moving without stopping! Since my parents were inviting us to a party with the whole family, I decided to calm his mood by taking him to the park for a breath of fresh air.

On the way back, I stopped at the supermarket and was just selecting some fruits, when suddenly the lights went out, and people started shouting: "Fire, Fire." Needless to say, I rushed outside and kept my self control with my son in my arms who was putting both hands against his ears, as if the noise or awful smell was disturbing him.

Since I was not feeling well myself, I decided to go straight to my parents, who were expecting us for dinner; and while we were sitting in the train, my son spent the forty minutes gesticulating a lot instead of sleeping. On our arrival, when my son saw my parents, he was staring at them, trying to make himself understood by shaking his head and his body, before suddenly twitching his arms, smacking his lips, jerking his head and his eyes. He stayed like that for ten minutes at least, and also had trouble breathing. I was unable to move and was mesmerized by my son's expression; he no longer looked like a baby, but like a serious adult transfixed by the fear!

When the doctor came five minutes after the attack, my son was still "weird" and very "white and blue," I should say. His temperature was higher than usual. After having an injection from the doctor, he was calm, but perspiring a lot. He slept for 9 hours without moving! I was not at all acquainted with this illness and was scared by this attack. It was the first one that I had seen.

Ten months later, he had his second seizure; and, this time, I was not afraid for his life, but still mesmerized by his dreadful, frightful expression. My little angel was looking devilish; and the funny part of this was that we were staying at a holy city well known for its healing powers!

Now, my son is 18 years old, and he still has seizures despite the anti-epileptic drugs; but I can say that he is living well with his illness and looks like anyone else. He has gained his friends' support by accepting the fact that he has epilepsy, and never complains about it. He acts with a certain fatalism that allows him to be himself and to keep his own personality; even if, sometimes, he looks like someone really weird and scary to people who are seeing him have a seizure for the first time.

He has always had a lot of freedom; he took public transportation by himself since he was 6 years old, and I let him do all kinds of sports in which he succeeds extremely well. Also my son maintains his self-confidence and is very optimistic.

4

Mother When my daughter was sixteen months old, she had meningitis. Although she had a number of seizures in the hospital, I never witnessed them. Her electroencephalogram was not normal, however, and for years I lived with the fear that she would develop seizures. I breathed a very large sigh of relief when she was nine and the neurologist told us that the annual check-ups were no longer indicated because she was doing so well.

While on a family vacation, when she was 13, she complained of headache and soon thereafter had a major seizure. Her body was rigid, there was twitching of the left arm and leg, she was disoriented and the first seizure was followed by four others. In between, she slept and could not be awakened. I have never been as frightened as I was on that day. At first I thought that she might die but as the seizures subsided, I realized that her life and ours would never be quite the same again.

Throughout the ensuing years, she has been well controlled with medication. Her seizures occur only when she is falling asleep. She begins to talk in a high pitched voice, the left side of her face twitches, then her arm and finally her leg twitch. They last less than a minute. She falls asleep and cannot be awakened.

Although I feel she has been fortunate that her seizures are not more severe or frequent, I am left with a sadness that I realize will always be there.   *56*

5a

Mother A slight moan turned my head to the attention of my son. One look at his face told me he was going to have a seizure. How did I know? The change in his eyes told you he had no control over what was about to happen. His hand came forward, and his arms curved in almost a fetal manner, his body became rigid, and his legs became unsteady as though they refused to hold his weight.

There are two instances that I can relate. He set aside one day to work in the attic, looking for items he had stored from years gone by. He had a great time finding things that he had forgotten were there. After an hour or two, he realized he had better give up since his wife would be home from work and any more would have to be done another time. After putting the ladder away, he commented that he "did not feel too good." His father asked, "What's the trouble?" My son said, "I think I'm going to be sick." He became rigid and started to lose his balance. His eyes became glazed over and foam appeared at his mouth. His father grabbed him to keep him from falling; their bodies hurtled around the kitchen. My son is a strong man, 5 ft 11 inches tall and 220 lbs. His father is 5 ft 11 inches tall and about 240 lbs. And he had all he could to hold him up. My son coughed, showing distress at the mucous or foam that crowded his throat, his arms flailed in erratic movements, and his father held his knee out in chair like fashion so that he could have some support, some place to rest to keep him off of the floor. I rushed to wipe his mouth and he started to make moaning noises, strange sounds that made no sense at all for awhile and then became loving, saying how much he loved his Dad who was the one holding on to him at the time. I somehow knew that he was coming out of it.

Exhaustion hit all of us. My son for what he had just gone through, my husband from the battle of keeping his son from being hurt, the stress and strain of holding him up, and the heartache of knowing that was all he could do for him. He could not kiss it and make it better the way he could when he was small; all he could do was watch.

Immediately following this and other seizures my son has to stretch out on the bed since he is completely tired out. Sometimes he would fall asleep, but in about 10 or 15 minutes he has to urinate. He would have to go immediately to the bathroom. (I always wondered if there was some connection between his seizures and his kidneys.)

Once my son had an errand to do over at a local hospital. His father and I offered to drive him over since we had to be in the same area that day. He said wonderful. My son sat in back and we talked and chatted. For a moment there was silence. I looked back, thinking he had dozed. As soon as I looked, I knew he was starting to have a seizure. His face was expressionless and his eyes stared straight ahead. His face was pale, and he murmured quietly, "I'm going to be sick." He stiffened and moaned as though in pain. I reached back to feel his face in sympathy (the feeling of complete helplessness). His face was wet with perspiration. Foam (white) started coming from his mouth. His eyes were glazed and I knew he did not hear me; his left hand started to rub his face, with no control, rubbing it hard, very hard; he started to choke. I tried to wipe the foam from his mouth fearing he would choke on it but it did not seem to help. He started to pick up papers that were on the seat of the car. His motions were erratic. He started to sweat. His body was under a tremendous strain—it lasted for about fifteen minutes at least. Later on he said this was a "mini seizure." Not to me.

As a mother I can not help but wonder what this does to the rest of his body. The strain is that great. *54*

5b

Wife I first witnessed my husband having a seizure in July of 1982. It was a very hot day and we had both gone down to a beach, which was a short walk from his parents' house. We were not married at the time.

We were the only people on the beach. I had just come out of the water when he decided to go in. But before he made it into the water, he said that he felt sick and leaned to one side. He then began to shake violently. As a result of this shaking, he started to roll off of the blanket and onto the sand. I tried to keep him on the blanket as the sand was rather rocky but it was impossible. I had heard about seizures and knew what to do about them from numerous first aid courses I had taken. I had never seen anyone have a seizure before, but somehow it seemed as if I had. I wasn't prepared, however, when he began scooping up sand and rocks in his hands and putting them in his mouth. I was terrified that he would choke on a rock but when I yelled "stop!" he did stop. He then began to vomit and shortly after that "came to." When I was able to get him to sit on the blanket, I wet some towels in the water and wiped his sweaty, sandy body with them. He seemed O.K. with only a few minor scratches but said that he had a terrible headache. He didn't know what had happened to him so I explained the best I could.

We managed to walk back to his parents' house. When his father opened the door he had a look of terror on his face. He knew something was wrong. I told his father that I thought that his son had a convulsion. His father and mother immediately led him to his bedroom. They helped him to lie down on his bed, turned the air conditioner on, and put cool cloths on his forehead. His father called their family doctor and explained what happened. The doctor told us to take him down to the hospital immediately.

His father drove to the hospital. He was seen immediately in the emergency room. His condition was assessed and many doctors questioned me about what had happened. At first the doctors felt that he had simply suffered from heat exhaustion but they were unsure. From my explanation of what had happened they felt that he may have indeed had a seizure. He apparently had seizures before as a child but didn't have one in many years and at this time was not on any seizure medication. He was admitted to the hospital for observation but since it was a Friday afternoon, no tests could be performed until Monday.

I spent the weekend at his parents' house. By Saturday morning he felt fine and was up and about. On Monday an EEG was performed that revealed abnormal brain waves. As a result, the neurologist put him on medication for seizures.

Since then, he continues to have a seizure about once a month. At times they have been more frequent and at times less. He has been on various medications for them and is currently on two antiepileptic drugs. He sees his neurologist regularly. When he is going to have a seizure he will say to me, "Uh, can you help me, I don't feel good." He will be hunched over and all color will be gone from his skin. I try to steer him to the couch, bed or a sturdy chair to sit down. If this is not possible, I sort of brace him against a wall. His body is so rigid when he is in a seizure that it would be impossible to lie him on the floor without injuring him. He is also a very large man. As the seizure proceeds, he leans to the right, groans, drools and his eyes look glassy. As he begins to come out of a seizure he rubs his face with his hands hard and furiously. He speaks meaningless phrases and becomes affectionate towards me. It usually takes a good five to ten minutes before he completely recovers from a seizure and can speak coherently. When the seizure has ended he will say something to me such as "I guess I got sick." He is very tired afterwards and needs to go directly to bed.

We have been married for almost ten years now and live in an apartment. We do not have any children but hope to. He works part time as a security guard and I work full time as a day care teacher and part time in a laundromat. His seizures hinder him from finding full time work and finances for us are tight. I am used to him having seizures but they always catch me off guard and any immediate plans we may have before he has a seizure have to be postponed until he recovers. If he feels a seizure coming on we will avoid leaving home because it would be a catastrophe to us both if he had one in public. Strangers do not understand his seizures like I do and some well-meaning person may call an ambulance when it would not be necessary. I would say that my husband having epilepsy does make our lives a challenge but we are fortunate to have the closeness, love and support of each other as well as our families. *54*

6

Wife The first time I saw my husband have a convulsion, I wasn't sure at first what was happening—it wasn't at all "like on T.V."—it was a "slow motion" type of change until his whole body started convulsing. I felt a wave of fear for him and scared because although I knew he had epilepsy, I wasn't sure what to do! (And I'm a Registered Nurse.)

It lasted only about 2 minutes but seemed longer. I left him alone and in his post-ictal state he was very calm, did not act like anything happened although he was now on the floor. When I kept repeating "Are you alright? You've just had a seizure," he seemed dazed, confused and when he finally realized what had happened, he started to cry. And again, I wasn't sure why he was crying. He kept repeating "I don't want to go. I don't want to go."

I later learned that he always was taken to the hospital to have his blood drawn and he hated this routine. He still acts strange after a seizure saying things like "I want to go home" when he is already home.

He doesn't have a lot of convulsions; only when he's very sick with a fever (usually 5–7 days later) or he forgets his medication. But he still suffers from these "drop" attacks. I don't know what else to call them. After waking up either in the morning or after a long nap, his body just buckles under for a few seconds. I believe he loses consciousness for a few seconds and then it stops. But he has fallen onto things, dropped things or bumped into objects. I am very concerned that he may seriously hurt himself at work when this happens. It seems to occur 30–40 minutes after waking up and may happen once or twice in succession depending upon how tired he is.

I also get worried when I'm working and he's home with our two daughters. Our older one (13) understands, but the 5-year-old doesn't have a clue and I don't want her to get scared watching

Epilepsy in Our View

Daddy "shaking out of control." I send her out of the room, which makes her want to come back even more.

He doesn't really acknowledge these drop attacks. I get angry and frustrated because I think he *must* know when he falls, or drops something, but he makes excuses like "it slipped" or he lost his balance and *denies anything* is wrong when I've seen these little "spells" occur. If I ask him if anything happens at work, he says no. His secretary, however, tells me when she notices funny things. I'm not sure if it is all denial with him, or else he just won't admit that he knows what's happening, or maybe he doesn't really know? I tend to doubt that, though. *51*

7

Mother My son's seizures started at age 17. He would suddenly have a blank stare and then fall into a convulsion. After it stopped he would sometimes be sick to his stomach and then go into a deep sleep for about two hours. He complained of a headache after this.

Throughout the years, we thought he was ignoring us when we were having a conversation if he did not answer when spoken to. We are now aware that this was another form of seizure. He has told us he does have a warning but tries to fight it off.

From the time all this began he has gone from an easy-going person to one who is difficult to get along with. But we have noticed a big difference in him since the medication was changed. His eyes are clear (not heavy like they used to be) and he has an easier personality. He seemed to have seizures more often when he was under stress. We see him occasionally now as he lives by himself.

I hope this information is a help to you. We feel for the first time since all this started, that he has hope for the future.

8a

Husband My wife's seizures started about three years before our son was born and consisted of blank stares and inability to communicate, lasting about 30 seconds.

Shortly after our son was born, my wife burned her hand in a frying pan. Her hand lay in the pan burning and she felt no pain. Over time, she started showing increased seizure activity. I became fearful of her dropping the baby and tried to get her to seek medical aid.

It was difficult to get a diagnosis. But finally it came through. Medication helped, but she burned herself again when our son was around three. Also, she started having blackouts when driving. I was always dreading a phone call that she and our son had a serious accident.

Personally, it was an uncomfortable time. Just imagine fearing your wife might die and leave you alone to raise a son by yourself. And the medical profession could do so little. I was helpless during her seizures and embarrassed at times in the presence of others. I'm so glad something was able to help her at last.   *48*

8b

Mother At the start of a seizure, her eyes would have a "vacant" look, as though she was in a trance. Her jaw would move as though she were chewing, and she would swallow quite frequently during the spell. She would want to be held closely until the seizure passed, a matter of a few minutes. When she came out of it, she would not recall what had happened. Unless she had suffered an injury during the seizure, she would resume her normal activity in a short period of time. *48*

8c

Son When I was a child, witnessing one of my mother's seizures was a frightening experience, but as I aged, I became used to them. When my mother had a seizure or "spell" as I referred to it she would, without warning, almost lose consciousness but would still be able to stand reasonably on her own. Her seizures generally lasted under a minute or up to a minute and a half but no longer. While her seizures were so short and mild, there was no warning or tell-tale signs to alert anyone that she was about to have one. She just did, making her choice to give up her license valid. If she had a seizure when I was present, she would usually look right at me and smile with a somewhat dumbfounded look on her face. Her mouth would move sporadically in a side-to-side chewing fashion and she would "furrow" her eyebrows as if she was concentrating. As I mentioned before, when I was younger this would scare me, but as I got older, I found the look on her face was quite amusing and it was hard not to laugh. I found that when she was having a seizure, if I said "Mom" repeatedly, she would look right at me. From this I assumed that it did not affect her hearing.

After my mother came out of a seizure she would usually not even know that she had one unless someone told her or she had fallen and hurt herself if she was alone. After she was fully aware and out of the seizure she usually needed to sit down and rest for a

Seizure Descriptions

minute since she was exhausted, and sometimes requested something to drink to "wet her whistle."

I wish I could be more specific about my observations but her symptoms were so mild that if you didn't know she was having a seizure you probably wouldn't even notice unless she fell or dropped something like a shopping bag. *48*

9a

Sister My brother asked that I write to you describing my feelings about his epilepsy.

When he was first diagnosed, I was a little girl and did not understand what was happening. I was frightened that my little brother was sick with this strange disease that made him do strange things. I believe that I must have been somewhat embarrassed when he had a seizure in public.

For many years his seizures were under control and I ignored the fact that he had epilepsy. But when I was about 18 years old, my father stopped my brother's medication and he had a convulsion. I then realized that my brother was not cured and he would have to live with epilepsy for the rest of his life.

When the seizures started again, I was frightened for my brother's welfare. I felt helpless because there was nothing I could do and I was angry that this had to happen to him. Each time my brother has a seizure in my presence, or a seizure when we speak on the telephone, I am afraid that he will not come out of it. When he discusses the medical problems he experiences because of the drugs and the seizures, I become very upset and wish that sheer willpower would cure him. It hurts me to see him shake because of the drugs and it upsets me that his balance is off.

This winter I was very proud of him because he took up skiing. He persisted on the bunny slope and finally was able to go with the rest of his family to the more advanced slopes. This to me is a great accomplishment which takes courage.

I guess the feeling I always carry with me is that of helplessness because there is nothing I can do to restore his health.   *41*

9b

Son I am 7 years old. My daddy has epilepsy. I feel sad when I see him have a seizure. It looks like he's getting stiff. When he has a seizure, I hold his hand until the seizure is over. I sort of feel scared when he has a seizure.   *41*

9c

Wife My husband has had epilepsy as long as I've known him (over 22 years). I have seen 2 convulsions—both in the middle of the night. I was awakened by him thrashing around and foaming at the mouth. It lasted around 10 minutes, and then I noticed his eyes rolled back into his head, his arms and legs got rigid and finally he fell into a deep sleep. When he awoke the next morning, he had a terrible headache.

I have witnessed countless small seizures. He will be staring absentmindedly into the air for a few seconds, then his head will turn to the right and his right hand will start trembling for about 1 minute. Then he'll snap out of it, shake off the effects of the seizure and continue to do what he was doing prior to the seizure.   *41*

Seizure Descriptions

9d

Student The first time I saw my teacher have a seizure, I was a freshman, and it was scary. He told us that he was an epileptic and he had seizures about 5–10 times a day.

When he is going have a seizure he tells us. He said that he can hear himself talking. Then he turns his head to the right and lifts his right arm to a 90 degree angle. And then he revolves to the right. It lasts about 10–15 seconds.

The second time I saw him have a seizure, I laughed. I felt bad later. Kids in my shop class and I made some songs about it. But now I feel bad about it and try to help him or make it easier for him so he won't have to get nervous.   *41*

9e

Student Epilepsy or any other physical or mental disability does not bother me at all. On the first day of school as a freshman in high school, my shop teacher explained to us that he had epilepsy, how it affects him and what happens.

I had already been exposed to epilepsy. A family member of mine has it severely. This has helped me to accept it. But I often wonder, what does a person think or feel while having a seizure? What does it feel like to live with this disease, and how do others view you? There really is no need to criticize a person with a handicap. When you think of it, it doesn't make sense.   *41*

9f

Student The first time I saw my teacher have a seizure I wasn't very afraid or puzzled. He had explained it beforehand, so I knew what to expect. I have accepted it and it doesn't bother me.

When he is about to have a seizure he tells us. If he is sitting down he will stand up. His head goes to the right and sometimes he starts to shake. After the seizure ends he goes back to what he was doing before. *41*

9g

Student The first time I saw my teacher having a seizure I wasn't afraid or worried because it was already explained to me. Even so, whenever I see him having a seizure, I walk away from him until he stops having it.

I don't think there is anything wrong with it. *41*

9h

Student When I first saw my teacher have a seizure, I thought man this guy must have a screw loose.

When he is going to have a seizure I can tell because he just starts to blank out. Then his head turns and his nerves get jumpy. When it's all over, he comes to as if he has just woken up. *41*

9i

Student The first time I saw my teacher have a seizure I looked at him surprised because I didn't know what was going on with him. I thought he was making funny faces, but then I got scared. When he is going to have a seizure, he tells you, so you can wait a little longer and look the other way. When he has it, it's like he is not here, and when it is over, he starts talking to you.   *41*

9j

Student The first time I saw my teacher have a seizure, I was afraid. I did not know how or what he was going to do during the seizure. Even though I was told he had epilepsy and had seizures very often, I didn't know what was going to happen or how he was going to react. I felt bad the first time I saw him because I wanted to help, but couldn't.

Before he has a seizure he stops whatever he's doing and has an uncomfortable look on his face. He sometimes tells us to get away from him. Then he slowly turns his head to the side and looks like he is in another world. Once the seizure is over, he blinks and has a look of exhaustion on his face. He then tries to get back to what he was doing, but most of the time he doesn't remember.   *41*

9k

Student The first time I saw my teacher have a seizure I was scared, because I didn't know what to do. Every time before having a seizure, he tells us to go away and not to look at him. During the seizure I always go away, I really don't look at him. And when the seizure is over, he's in another world until he's back to normal again.   *41*

Student The first time I saw my teacher have a seizure it frightened me because I was about 2 or 3 feet from him and he just missed hitting me with his hand.

During his seizures his head moves to the right and he has no idea what he's doing. He also sticks his right hand out and starts spinning around. Just before, he begins he tells the person closest to him "to move away."

At the end of the seizure he practically does not remember a thing.   *41*

Student The first time I saw my teacher have a seizure I was afraid. I had never known anyone with epilepsy and I had never seen anyone have a seizure before.

Before he has a seizure he will blank out. He won't answer anyone or talk to anyone. While he is having a seizure his head turns to the right and sometimes he will move a few steps. After he has a seizure he shakes it off and gets back to what he was doing before. But sometimes he will forget what he was doing and move on to something else.   *41*

Seizure Descriptions

9n

Student The first time I saw it I felt nothing because I knew a kid that has it. I knew him for a month because his parents like to move. He was a cool kid. *41*

9o

Student When I first saw my teacher have a seizure I was kind of afraid. I had never seen anyone have a seizure before. Now it doesn't bother me at all.

Before he has a seizure he can't really concentrate on anything. During the seizure he turns his head to the side and kind of takes little steps or just turns around in a circle and stares into space. After the seizure he is very tired for a minute and usually yawns. *41*

10

Mother The first seizures I saw my son have were mild. He would stare into space and appear to be far, far away. He wouldn't answer when we talked to him. In a short time, a minute or less, he'd be back with us and never know they had occurred.

The first convulsion I saw took place on the patio. As far as I could see, there was no warning. We were talking and I was sewing. I went into the house to get a fresh spool of thread and when I came out he was on the ground. His back was arching and his head was rolling and thrashing about. We placed something soft (a towel, I think) around his head so he wouldn't hurt himself. This lasted for two or three minutes. When it was over he didn't know what had happened, but he was very tired. Exhausted, I would say. He lay down and slept the greater part of the day.

We have begged him to pace himself, but either he is unable or unwilling to do so. We love him very much, but find it hard to understand him. He's driven, but otherwise a warm, loving and caring person.

11a

Mother Our daughter's seizures have never been predictable, but once a seizure starts, it follows a pattern to some extent, but varies in length and intensity. Usually without warning, she begins to stare into space and says "wait, wait, wait, wait, wait" getting increasingly urgent in her expression. After saying "wait" she says no more, but the tension builds up in her body. She sucks her cheeks between her teeth and begins to chew on her tongue and on the inside of her mouth until it bleeds. If she chews her lips, they swell up as if badly bruised and sometimes she clamps her teeth together. While she is moving her mouth, she sometimes steps on one foot, then the other from side to side—sort of rocking. Other times, she backs up; several times she has stepped backwards off steps and has fallen. If she is holding something, it drops as her hands tense into fists, or contort as if in spasm, or as she rubs her thumbs repeatedly against her index fingers.

Her whole body seems tense and her skin seems cool and moist at the end of a seizure. I think her whole body perspires. After the seizure, she is stunned and vague for a short time, 2 to 5 minutes, then she converses hesitantly for a few minutes. Later she does not seem to remember anything that has happened during the half hour, or so, after the seizure. She feels nervous and tired and wants to sleep, often for an hour or more.

Her seizures started very mildly when she was about 12. She looked up at the ceiling and blinked her eyes. It seemed to happen when our children were together. I remember nudging my husband to notice this behavior. We discussed it and decided to say nothing to her, but to give her more attention, thinking her strange blinking was a bid for attention.

Back then, we called her seizures "spells." Soon the blinking stopped and she began to have "spells" in which she lost touch with reality. She stood or sat still as if dazed and would say something that had no meaning. Most of what she said was so irrelevant that when the "spell" was over, I could not remember what it was.

When she was in high school, we began the odyssey of endless doctors, psychiatrists, tests, and personality profiles. The results were all similar and most doctors said the brain wave tests showed some abnormalities, but not enough to call it epilepsy. When the seizures worsened, the abnormalities increased and the verdict became epilepsy. She was relieved to have her problem given a name so she no longer felt she was "crazy" and "alone." *37*

11b

Sister My sister's seizures have increased in severity over the years. When she first began having them, I was away at school. At first, I didn't realize she was having them. She would say something strange but then quickly return to the conversation.

Now she begins her seizures by saying "Wait, wait, wait, wait." She begins to rock a bit, clench her hands, and twist her mouth. I try to remain calm, but feel myself tense up. I try to make her comfortable, rub her back, and just be there for her when the seizure is over. She appears somewhat dazed when she is no longer seizing. I have asked her if she is alright and she usually answers in the affirmative. I don't mention the seizure, as we both know she has had another one.

I grieve for her predicament. Each time it happens, I hope it will be the last and that some medication or other remedy can be found to relieve her of this difficult handicap. *37*

11c

Friend I have witnessed quite a few of my friend's seizures due to the fact that I work with her every day. The most common type of seizure that she has starts with her saying "wait, wait, wait." She stares straight ahead, her cheeks cave in and she chews the inside of her mouth. Both of her hands clench together. Her left hand usually is different from her right, meaning the middle finger of her left hand is usually over the index finger. Her right hand is clenched in a fist. This usually lasts a couple of minutes. Then, she will let out a deep breath and her hands will drop. She will look around. I call her name and she will turn her head to whoever calls her name. She is still incoherent. A couple minutes go by and we begin asking her questions such as "Who am I?" and "Where are you?" Her responses are different. Her speech is sometimes mumbled and does not make any sense and sometimes she will know who I am or where she is. We keep talking to her and judge by her answers when she has come out of seizure. There are times she wants to get up and our boss commands her to sit down. She *always* does what he says due to the tone of his voice.

I really can't remember the first time I saw her have a seizure, but I can and *will never forget* one of the big seizures she had in a restaurant. We had to dial 911 and off to the hospital we went!   *37*

11d

Friend Just before my friend's seizures occur she sometimes gets very quiet or stares for a few seconds. Unless you are looking directly at her, however, you would not see this. Very often there is no significant difference.

During the seizure, you will usually hear the words "wait, wait" repeated several times until they are run together and mumbling starts. Chewing of the inside of her mouth is prevalent during each seizure. Her eyes appear to be very dilated and staring occurs. She may appear to be looking for something, move furniture, rearrange cushions/pillows, etc. and lift items up to look under them. This aspect of "looking for something" doesn't occur in each episode.

The actual "end" of the seizure is the most confusing part in my opinion. In other words, it is sometimes hard to tell exactly when she is back on track. Many times it appears she is functioning normally only to find out 10–20 minutes later she doesn't recall anything that was said or done during that time period.

The first time I saw a seizure it was surprising but not frightening. The seizures back then were quite different than the seizures now with only one common factor—the repetition of "wait, wait" has continued as long as I have known her (over 20 years). The seizures I witnessed back then were a lot faster and much more vocal. After the initial "wait, wait" she might strike up a conversation totally unrelated to anything that was going on. This usually brought a lot of raised eyebrows in our dorm at college.   *37*

12a

Friend In July, we had this little party at work. It was from 4:30 P.M. til 6:00 P.M. and people could come and look at our artwork and jewelry and potteries. Well I got there at 5:30 pm and was looking for my friend and other people. We were talking about her mother coming over and her other friend would be there soon.

I went to sit down and she sat down also. She got some grapes and crackers. I heard this whine, then a loud cry and I said to myself that it must be my friend. I went over to see what was happening and I saw her face was red and she was shaking. Her eyes were looking up into the ceiling and she was pushing her mother away while her mother was trying to hold her. All that time her face changed from red to a lighter gray/blue and I freaked out. I felt like crying. I hadn't seen anyone in a long, long time have a seizure. I walked away because I felt so bad, since I couldn't do anything for her.

I came back and I saw her just slipping off the chair onto the floor and she was more quiet now. I was still worried about her. She was still lying on the floor and she looked like she had just seen a ghost. I was upset for the rest of the night. She said she didn't know she had fallen on the floor or didn't remember me giving her a drink. She was out of it for a half hour.

12b

Mother When my daughter was 9 months old she had a high temperature. Her father picked her up because she was crying. While he was holding her in his arms—I still recall the incident—she started to shake. I immediately called the pediatrician and was told that

Seizure Descriptions

this was a febrile convulsion. I was instructed to give her cold compresses.

When she was 11 years old she had her first big seizure while we were at a family gathering in a park. She had no fever; however, she was experiencing her first menstrual period. Everyone was quite anxious and concerned.

The most recent seizure that I witnessed occurred at her job during an open house. I was standing near her and noticed that her eyes were blinking. While she was in a sitting position, she stopped and went into a convulsion. I caught her and someone else came to help because she was too heavy. All the guests stopped what they were doing and, of course, they were frightened. Yet no one panicked.

13

Mother When I describe my son's life with epilepsy, I think of what he has been able to accomplish, and only think of the epilepsy as a very small part of an enormous picture.

Let me first describe the seizures my son has experienced. He started having convulsions when he was 8 months old. He had an extremely high fever and a convulsion occurred. He had been sleeping when I heard noises in his room. He was gasping for air. His body was stiff. I thought for sure he was dying. We rushed him to the hospital. He was placed in cold packs for what seemed hours. It is hard to remember all that happened that evening—I just remember feeling he was going to die. He was only 8 months old! His fever finally broke. He was admitted, put on medication and put into an oxygen tent. He was in the hospital for three days. Then, he was released with a clean bill of health.

I was only 18 years old. I knew my son had been dangerously ill, but he was healthy again. I pushed the convulsion to the back of my mind and rarely thought about it again. Everything was normal, I felt, and I did not have to worry anymore.

Later, he started having small seizures. These were very mild and if you did not realize what was happening, you would have thought he was just daydreaming. He would smack and lick his lips, grind his teeth slightly and stare off into space. After a period of 5 to 10 minutes, he would return to normal and be extremely tired.

As time went by, he had big seizures. These were quite severe. His body would shake in erratic movements. He would make sounds and bite his tongue. He would fall on the ground if he were standing. Sometimes he would have 1 a week, sometimes 3 or 4 a day.

As a high school senior, he played nose guard for his football team and was an excellent team player. His teammates all knew of his condition and watched out for him. I only remember him having one very mild seizure at a game. The offensive line was in. He was on the sidelines. By the time the defensive line was sent back in, he was fine. He was sent back into the game and never missed a play. My fondest memory of my son playing football is one I really missed seeing. The opposing team was going for a field goal. If they made this play, his team would be the loser. I really was not paying attention to the final play. It was raining and cold. The game was about over. All of a sudden, the crowd roared. Over the loud speaker I heard something about my son. His sister was screaming. I could not hear what happened. Finally, after an endless minute I heard he had stopped the attempt. He made the play which saved the game for his team! His will to succeed has never failed him.

When he went to a local community college, he continued to have seizures on an irregular basis. Shortly after his graduation from high school, I received a call at work. He had been in another automobile accident. He had hit the back end of a van while having a seizure. His car was damaged, but luckily nobody was hurt. The police took his license at the scene. He has never tried to get it back again.

I wish I could tell the world what a caring, affectionate, courageous person he is. He loves people and most people who know him love him and miss him when he is not around. Epilepsy has caused him a lot of pain and heartache, but it has also made him strong. There are many diseases which affect our young people. All disorders involving young children are devastating and heart breaking. No matter what, these children are brave and strong. They are all natural fighters. They are all winners in a very special way. There is a song I especially love which reminds me of my son and all these children who suffer from illness. They are all my heroes, they are all "Wind Beneath My Wings."

14a

Mother My son was 14 years old. He appeared lethargic and was asleep on the couch when I returned home from work. This was after a football practice and we attributed the sleepiness to that. We discovered later that football practice included head bangs!

We didn't detect anything more unusual at that particular time but right after that he was experiencing hand and arm tremors and was dropping his shoes out of his hands in the morning while preparing for school. Then one morning we heard a crash from upstairs and our introduction to epilepsy began. It was difficult for us to face what was going on. This was a trying time at home for us because of the loss of a child two years before.

I was overwhelmed, angry, depressed, frightened, and desperately trying to hold onto family and job and maintain composure. His stepfather was angry and panicky, and was at wits end (as I) to sort out this latest crisis. What was a seizure? What was not? The years to follow were marked by poor communication, tension and turmoil.

For my son there were many crashes to the floor or in the shower. There were police incidents, work related accidents, and school calling to have him brought home. There were many losses— of jobs, driver's license, and friends. There were some unkind professionals lacking sympathy and attempts to exclude our involvement in treatment. There were many years of denial on his part and frustration and helplessness on ours.

It wasn't until he began treatment with a neurologist at a hospital that we felt we were being listened to, not judged, and that he began to receive specialized and caring treatment.

The never knowing and the unpredictable behaviors and watching your child lose his life goals and skills, while he struggles and is determined to become independent—this has been a painful experience for us.

Our faith and trust in God, our support of each other and the support and help of the hospital staff and the local epilepsy society has been and continues to be our strength and hope. *30*

14b

Sister My first reaction to seeing my brother have a seizure was to run the other way, which I did. He had a seizure on the school bus one morning. When the other kids saw this they started laughing, thinking he was joking around. When I saw this, I ran out of the bus to get the nurse. I should have stayed.

After a while, I got used to the seizures, but the anger stayed the same. Part of me felt guilty for being healthy but part of me was angry as a teenager because he got all the attention. Now as an adult I realize how hard his life has been and still is. The guilt is still there. The feeling of being helpless gets stronger as he gets older because he gets more and more distant from me.

The only anger I feel now is the fact that he just won't let any of us help him. But in a way I can't blame him because he is trying to keep some independence. *30*

15a

Cousin The first time I saw my cousin have a seizure we were at the beach. She suddenly got quiet, which was very unlike her. I asked her if she wanted to get a pizza. She didn't answer so I asked her again and she responded with "Where's my thing?" I said "What thing?" "You know my thing—the thing I drive," she said. "What are you talking about?" I asked and then I looked at her. Her face had the look of total confusion but her eyes looked blank. I thought "Oh my God, she's having a seizure now! What do I do?" I kept talking to her, asking her questions but for 2 minutes all she could say was "Where's my thing? (car). What do I do now? Where's my mother? What are we doing here? How'd we get here?"

I knew she was coming out of it when she asked "What just happened to me? I had a seizure didn't I?" I said yes, it lasted about 2½ minutes. She said she had a massive headache and asked for a painkiller. Then she wanted to go home and go to sleep.

Those 2½ minutes seemed like an hour. She seemed like a child asking the same questions over and over and couldn't understand the answers. I felt very frustrated because there was nothing I could do to make it pass faster.

15b

Friend From what I have seen, my friend has a very mild type of seizure. In many cases I've looked at her seizures as staring spells. She tends not to know what's going on during the spell. At first she continues talking, but then she looks like she's beginning to space out. She also keeps asking "What" and at times she continues to walk around as though she knows where things are. At times she is able to snap out of it.

15c

Mother In the following paragraphs I have explained to my daughter what happens when she has seizures. I am legally blind, therefore I could not write it myself.

Fifty percent of the time before she has a seizure she complains of a headache, or she tells me it's cold and she gets goose-bumps, or chills. She also seems fidgety or hyper. A lot of the time she will come out of a different room in the house, look at me and say "I had one of those things," meaning a seizure. She asks "What did I do?" or "What happened?" When she comes completely out of her state of confusion, she'll tell me "I had a seizure, what did I do?" It's as if she blocks out the word seizure until she is totally out of the seizure and confusion.

During a seizure she usually continues doing just what she was doing before the seizure began. For example, if she is eating, she continues to eat. Sometimes she will twirl her food with her fork a little, but she will finish her meal, sometimes eating at a faster pace.

Seizure Descriptions

During one of her seizures she was baking pies. She was completely "out of it." She could not answer my questions but she continued reading the recipe and taking the ingredients from the cupboard and refrigerator, measuring and mixing the ingredients. She totally prepared the pies! There was already one pie in the oven and the timer went off. She tested the pie and removed it from the oven, and then she placed the other two pumpkin pies in the oven. She looked at me and said "I'm going to bed." (She was still in a state of confusion.)

Sometimes during a seizure she will say "I have to get to a thing," meaning bathroom, and is usually able to find it on her own no matter where we are. During a seizure she looks like she's "on cloud nine." Her facial expression is very blank and her eyes seem glassy and staring. The seizures can last from two to ten minutes; seventy-five percent of the time they are three to four minutes in length. The state of confusion after the seizure lasts between ten to fifteen minutes, although half of the time there is no confusion; it's as if she just snaps right back to reality. Sometimes after a seizure, usually when there is a "state of confusion," she will become cold and very tired and will take a two hour nap. This may only happen once a month (she has six to ten seizures per month). After each seizure she always complains of a headache and takes a painkiller.

The first few times I saw my daughter "space out" I didn't realize they were seizures. She would just stand in the middle of the room and stare blankly. I thought she was kidding around.

16

Wife The first time I saw my husband have a seizure was at a restaurant. I had known him for about 7 years and the seizure really bothered me. He dropped his fork, smacked his lips and had a "funny looking" expression. I asked him if everything was all right and he just kept staring. He would never confide in me exactly what his illness was. It wasn't until I filled a prescription for him that I confronted him.

The first few years of our marriage were not significant in relation to his seizures. After about eight years, things started to worsen. It seemed like every time we went out, he'd have a seizure. He always felt the urge to urinate and would pull down his fly and expose himself. He'd start to take off his shirt. My biggest fear was that this would happen when he was alone and that he'd get arrested. Who would believe him? At this time I told my children about their father's illness and explained to them what to do if they were alone with him and he began to seize.

As time went on, visits to various doctors seemed fruitless. They kept adjusting his medication—increasing one and decreasing the other. He became toxic once and was a "walking zombie." He started having big seizures. The stress was unbelievable. Whenever the phone rang and he was late coming home, I would panic. The phone calls to my place of employment sent me reeling. By the time I got to the phone, I could hardly breathe.

Prior to a seizure, he would either leave the room to hide or try to sit away from us. He would stare with a funny grin on his face. If spoken to he would say "No!!" no matter what was said to him. If he was holding something he would drop it. He would unbutton his shirt, undo his belt buckle and pull out his penis as if to urinate. After the seizure, he would rub his hands together, say something silly and fall asleep for a while.

He would never remember what he did during the seizure. He knew he must have done something when he realized his pants were unzipped. His speech would be incoherent for a couple of minutes after the seizure. He would get frustrated when trying to communicate.

Seizure Descriptions

17a

Mother I have been with my daughter many times while she was having a seizure. When it starts she has a faraway look on her face. She becomes pale and disoriented and her hand shakes. She seems to be weak and needs to sit and recover. This all happens in about five to ten minutes. Sometimes she becomes nauseated but quickly recovers without vomiting.

17b

Sister When I was asked to describe my sister's seizures, I recalled vividly one seizure I witnessed a year ago. My sister, myself and my son were on the floor in my TV room playing a game. Suddenly she stopped what she was doing. I looked over at her and noticed she was very pale. She had a blank, spacey look on her face and her hands were trembling. She had difficulty getting up off the floor. She finally made it to the couch, but she did not look any better and her hands were still trembling. She ended up in the bathroom and threw up. After that she went to bed for the evening. She looked much better the next day.

17c

Sister I have been with my sister on several occasions when she has had seizures. To my eyes, the onset was subtle and I wasn't fully aware that the seizure had begun until I noticed that she was not engaged in the surrounding activity. She had an expression that was both pained and frightened and seemed to be caught in a freeze-frame. After the seizure, which lasted only 20–30 seconds, she was weak and upset, as if she were unnerved by the experience. Everyone else was upset for her as well and tried to calm her and reassure her.

18a

Brother I have observed my brother's seizures ranging from "space outs" to severe seizures. The first time I saw a bad seizure was quite alarming. My brother was shaking and foaming at the mouth. This type of seizure only lasted a minute or two. It was really scary to see. After this type of seizure, my brother would be very dazed and not remember what happened.

I have also observed milder seizures or "space outs." When he has a space out my brother will stare blankly into space. When this happens, he will not respond to any verbal communication. During another type of seizure, his muscles and face tense up. After about a minute of this my brother will return to normal. During the time his muscles tense up he appears to have no awareness of what is going on around him.

18b

Mother When my son had his first seizure it came as quite a shock to me. It happened during Christmas school vacation just two weeks before his fifteenth birthday. It was in the morning and he was still in bed. I was in the kitchen. I heard this crash from his bedroom overhead. I rushed upstairs to find him on the floor. He had fallen out of bed and was quite rigid, with a lot of shaking and foaming at the mouth.

I was alone at the time, so I hurried down the stairs to call 911. When I went back upstairs he was starting to get up although he was still in a daze. I wanted to get him back into bed, but at that point he started to go down the stairs and I couldn't stop him, so I helped him hoping we both wouldn't take a fall. When we got down, he went into the bathroom and immediately locked the door.

Very soon the emergency unit arrived and after many pleas to open the door, they finally had to remove the whole lock to get him out. He was taken to the hospital by ambulance and remained there until he was well enough to come home where he slept for most of the afternoon.

18c

Teacher A student of ours had 3 seizures during a 50-minute sports class where he was playing floor hockey. The first one occurred while he was playing hockey and running. He started to fall. His face became contorted and he clenched the hockey stick so tightly that we could not get it out of his hands. He was shaking and trembling. We eased him to the floor. The seizure lasted almost 2 minutes. He was perspiring a great deal. It was much worse than other seizures he had in the gym.

The second seizure occurred while he was walking across the gym to ask if he could reenter the game. This seizure consisted of turning his head to the side and staring for a while.

The third seizure occurred while he was goaltending and was fairly active. He turned his head to the side, stared and started to shake, but he did not fall down. He did seem much more confused and disoriented afterwards than he usually was after a seizure.

19

Mother This is about my son. His seizures came about because of a head injury 12 years ago. The first seizure scared me to pieces. I had never seen a seizure before and the one good thing was that he was in bed when it happened.

One day my son and I were riding on the highway. We were chatting and then he became quiet. I looked over and he had started to have a seizure. I got off the highway and drove to the local fire department and they took him to the clinic.

Another time he was in the kitchen after dinner doing the dishes. We heard the water running but thought nothing of it. My husband went into the kitchen and discovered him having a seizure. His cheek was resting on the hot water faucet and his hands were in the hot water. The ambulance took him to the clinic. His hands and cheek were badly burned. I brought him home that night.

The last seizure I saw him have was about 5 years ago. He was in the hospital where they were determining about the possibility of an operation to help control his seizures. He and I were sitting in his room chatting and watching T.V. All of a sudden his eyes glazed over and slowly a big seizure began. Because they had been reducing his medication the seizure was quite severe.

I realize that perhaps my own feelings during the seizures were not described fully. One reason for this is that when he had the seizures I knew it was up to me to find the correct help as soon as possible. I feel that life has been terribly unfair to him and I regret that each seizure takes a little more away from him. I also feel sorry for myself, because he will never be the son he would have been without seizures.

20

Mother With my son, it is extremely difficult to determine if there is a warning sign. He has not had a seizure in two years. Prior to that incident he had not had one in five years. He is still on two anti-seizure medications. When he was exhibiting active seizures, he often complained of a headache. He would point to the center of his head.

21

Father It's New Year's Day, 28 years ago and I was awakened by screams from my wife. Something was wrong with our youngest child who was one year old. I ran into the bedroom and found him gagging. He was evidently having a seizure; my instinct was to pull his tongue out with my fingers, which I did accomplish. As I was doing this, my wife was calling the emergency number for the police department. My other three children, ages 3, 5, and 8 were looking on. The police and fire departments arrived and after emergency first aid rushed him to a local hospital.

He was admitted, tests were done, and a neurologist was sent in to evaluate the situation. We were told that he definitely had a grand mal seizure. He was put on anticonvulsant medication and he didn't have another seizure until a year later when he had another grand mal seizure. He also became hyperactive and destroyed things at home if not watched carefully.

He was evaluated at several local hospitals and given IQ tests. One neurologist told us that he was retarded. He had another test by a leading pediatric neurologist and his staff and we were told that he was not retarded. It was discovered that the anticonvulsant drug was causing the hyperactivity, or at least making it worse. He was taken off the medication at that time.

When a new drug came out he was put on that along with another drug. He soon developed a skin allergy to one of the drugs and had to be taken off. He would have many seizures over the years until another new drug came out. These seizures included jerking and looking out into space. Only once since he was put on this drug has he had any type of seizure. This was when he was 14 years old and was developing chicken pox. He is now being tapered off one of the medications and will be maintained on the other.

My son is now 18 years old, has his driver's license, works an average of 20–25 hours/week and will graduate from high school next year. He has been a special needs student throughout his school years and for the past year he has been mainstreamed into some regular classes.

People with epilepsy can live normal lives like most people. They may have certain problems that other people don't understand and therefore more should be written so the public can understand.

22a

Mother My daughter's first seizure happened when she was six years old. Three of us were there. My daughter-in-law was frightened and ran to get her mom and call an ambulance. My eldest daughter and I picked her up off the floor and placed her on the bed. She sounded as though she was choking so I turned her head to the side. This was done by instinct. She was shaking all over. We could do nothing but stand and watch helplessly.

When the medics came they told us that we should have held her down. They said we should have placed something between her teeth, but the seizure had come on without warning. Her jaws were clamped together so tight that we would have had to break her teeth to do that. We talked to her to let her know that we were there. When she awoke she said that she could hear every word that was said, and asked us to let her sit up if it happened again. After that first seizure, we held her hands and let her sit up and talked to her. This made her less scared.

We went out the next day and found books and descriptions of epilepsy and learned all we could about medications and their side effects. She has had epilepsy, which by the way, was once called the illness of royalty, for twenty-five years now, in many forms. She has learned to accept the painful bruises, the split-open cuts and stitches as part of her life. By the way, we learned *never to place anything in her mouth or to hold her down.*

I can only stand by and support her and love her. I only wish that other people had more understanding and were not so afraid of epilepsy. *27*

22b

Sister My sister was injured 6 months before my wedding. She was struck by a motorcycle and left in a coma. Our family life was torn apart. When she came home, she had to wear a helmet because the bone was removed from the right side of her head. We did not postpone my wedding. She became part of everything. She did very well, but sometimes we resented all the attention she received. Sometimes we were ashamed of her seizures. They embarrassed us. Other times we felt guilty because she was never able to do all the things we could.

Now I look at her and see how many things in life she has missed. Life must be very hard for people with epilepsy, and sometimes very embarrassing and lonely. She has had this illness for twenty-five years, and has no one now but our mother. I love her and pray for help to come to her.   *27*

23

Mother When my son has a seizure, he turns his eyes to the right and stares. Often, he repeats a word like wow or oh, oh. He may also have severe cramps, and pushes in on his stomach. Then the cramps seem to stop, and his head tips forward and his right arm and leg jerk. This lasts about 15 seconds.   *26*

24

Wife My husband had his only convulsion about 31 years ago. This was three weeks after the birth of our daughter. He was referred to a neurologist and after much testing it was concluded that this was probably a one time episode caused by stress. We had just transferred to another state and he had changed jobs. We had a new baby to add to our family that already included two children under the age of three. It made good sense to attribute the seizure to stress and we were relieved temporarily.

However, a few months later, he started experiencing blackouts. They consisted of chewing and swallowing and not being responsive to anything that was going on around him. He never fell or had any physical symptoms other than the chewing. The blackouts would last usually less than a minute. He would be disoriented for a short time after some of these episodes.

About ten years ago, the blackouts changed. From his point of view, he was not experiencing any blackouts at work. While this was a welcome report, I noticed that he seemed to be experiencing them at about the same frequency while I was with him. We therefore concluded that he was probably still blacking out at work but was not remembering them. Chewing did not seem to be present. He would smile broadly and go through the process of trying to straighten anything that might be in reach. The duration continued to be brief.

I have noticed that he usually has a cluster of three seizures in a day. Often, but not always, the seizures are preceded by a bad headache. He always goes to the bathroom after one of these blackouts. Again he is disoriented for a short time afterwards. He used to have a fabulous memory but now it is average and on some days poor. After a day of blackouts, he will doze off to sleep in his chair in the evening. This is unusual for him.

Seven years ago, we decided that the stress of trying to appear as if all was well was not helping him. Since our children were all out of college, we decided it was time for a change of life style. He took early retirement and we became owners of a bed and breakfast. This has worked out well for both of us. I did notice that he was foggy a lot of the time and his quality of life was not what it should be. There were adjustments made in the amount of drug that he was taking. We found that the blackouts did not increase or decrease but he was feeling 100% better. He was seeing better (from bifocals to 20/20 vision without glasses), he was not staggering and bumping into things and he was not living in a fog all the time.

Overall, he is in excellent health and is feeling terrific except for the blackouts.

25a

Boyfriend The first time I saw my girlfriend have a seizure was roughly 3 years ago. We were driving home from college (with her in the front passenger seat and myself driving) and all of a sudden she became quiet. I asked her what was the matter. Then, she turned to me with a blank face and her mouth wide open. Suddenly, she started to "cringe up" and jerk violently. I put her seat belt on so she would not hurt herself. She was also biting her tongue and making a heavy "slurring" noise. This whole process lasted about 5 minutes. Afterwards, I brought her to the hospital. She did not remember what happened when she awoke at the hospital. After the seizure was over she fell asleep.

I never saw anybody have a seizure before or knew anybody with a seizure disorder. Obviously, I felt bad for her and hoped that she was all right. Witnessing someone have a seizure when you do not know what to expect is very scary.

25b

Mother The first time I saw my daughter have a seizure was 10 years ago. She was watching T.V. when I called her. She wasn't responding so I went to see her. At first I thought she was having a heart attack but realized something else was wrong because her body was jerking and she was making a slurring sound. I still didn't know what was wrong so I called for help. When the ambulance arrived she seemed to be tired and was sort of out of it. The ambulance driver indicated that she had a seizure. We took her to the emergency room at the hospital. They kept her overnight, ran tests and confirmed that she did have a seizure.

When she had her first seizure I had no idea what was happening. I was extremely scared and just wanted her to be fine. I had never seen anyone have a seizure and I had no idea what to do.

26

Friend The first episode occurred when my friend got up around 6:30 am and sat on the toilet. Shortly thereafter, as I was lying in bed awake, I heard a very loud, guttural animal sound and sat up in the bed. As the bathroom door was opened, I saw that she fell off the toilet and landed in between the vanity and bathtub. I ran into the bathroom. She was on her back with both hands brought up into her chest with claw-like features to her hands, eyes rolled back, teeth clenched, not really making the guttural noises any longer but more of a heavy breathing sound. She had blue lips. I turned her over to her right side and straddled her so that she would not hit any of her extremities on the vanity or the tub. There were jerking motions of all four extremities. The seizure probably lasted 90 seconds to 2 minutes. When she stopped, I tried to wake her but it seemed as if she were in a deep sleep. She was breathing evenly and her mouth was more relaxed and teeth had become unclenched. There was no urinary or stool incontinence.

Emergency Medical Technicians had arrived by this time (as I had called them before I even left the bed to go to her aid) and she gradually began to come around, I would say 2–3 minutes after the end of the seizure. She was very confused and was quite frightened to see herself on the floor with the two men staring down at her. She seemed to have slurred speech and was somewhat lethargic on first awakening and was assisted to a nearby chair. She was uncooperative, did not want to go to the hospital, would not lie on a stretcher and finally agreed to be carried down in a chair. This resulted in a 2 day admission at the local hospital.

The second episode happened approximately 1½ to 2 years later, off of medication. She was taking a nap in the early afternoon on a Friday night and our other roommate came into my bedroom. She (the other roommate) started to show me the clothes she had purchased that night and my friend heard her, got up and walked into my bedroom. Within 1–2 minutes while standing up she looked at me, put both of her arms straight out in front of her and started saying my name over and over. I knew that she was going to have another seizure. I managed to lie her down on the bed onto her right side and within seconds, she again had a seizure with all four extremities jerking, blue lips, teeth clenched, arms bent at the elbows, hands pulled up towards her chest, with the heavy breathing noises as mentioned above, again no incontinence of either urine or stool. This episode lasted maybe 1–2 minutes. She seemed to be in a deep sleep, again for 2–3 minutes and upon awakening, was confused, being more agitated than the first time. She even pushed away a female Emergency Medical Technician and was very uncooperative, saying that she wanted her mother to be called (whom she had told me earlier was shopping at a nearby mall and, therefore, could not be reached). She did not want to go to the hospital. She was finally convinced (with us begging and the other roommate in tears) to go to the local emergency room for further treatment.

She told me later on that she knew that she was going to have this second seizure and that is why she was calling my name.

27

Friend The first time I saw my friend have a seizure, he was in bed. There was no warning. He made guttural sounds and had spastic motions. The main thing I recall was that everything seemed to be in slow motion, although the actual duration was very short. Only a couple of minutes, I think. I was not nervous about it as he had prepared me and he was in no danger. He was sleepy afterward and had a severe headache for most of the day.

The seizure I think of most vividly was when he hit a window several stories above ground. No one was around. Later I saw how the window was broken. This seizure frightened me very much and illustrated to me how extremely serious they are. This was apparently a more serious seizure than the one I witnessed as he seemed more disoriented afterwards, and for quite a few days. He had not gone to pick up his pills. It seemed that the cause of the seizure was due to not taking his medication. This has happened before, though he is normally a very cautious and sensible man, I can only assume there is a strong emotional aspect to his reaction to his illness.

28a

Mother The first time I saw my daughter have a seizure I was somewhat frightened but remembered her husband saying to stay calm and to talk to her. She was visiting me and supposedly talking to her husband on the telephone. When I called her for dinner and she didn't respond I knew something was wrong. So I calmly kept talking to her until she hung up the phone. She was somewhat disoriented but slowly came around and was very upset because I saw her in that condition. I assured her that I loved her and it didn't change our relationship—it made me realize just how serious this disease can be and how it cripples one's independence.

28b

Sister My sister's seizures have been categorically filed under "petit mal" but the one, two or three minute "suspension in time" she goes through is horrifying to watch. All her seizures that I observed, now thinking about it, begin with her coughing lightly, almost like she has a "tickle" in her throat that she can't quite clear. The next moment she is only physically present—her mind is clearly not present.

My first reaction is that she not inadvertently hurt herself; if she had anything in her hand I would try to take it away. One surprising element in this is that she would respond to my endeavor to "make her safe" by making guttural sounds which communicated to me that she wanted me to leave her and her belongings alone. The most frustrating and longest moments are waiting until she "comes back around." Knowing she will not harm herself, you can only sit and feel helpless until she "returns to the present." For the outsider a few seconds do seem like an eternity. She will always "return" stating: "I feel so tired." That is when I know she is back with us. She would get up and go lie down. Naturally, for the onlooker, you are thrilled she's "back" but I also dread having to let her know she'd had a seizure because of her disappointment in their occurrence. In spite of that, she always tells us to let her know so that she could keep track and regulate her medicine. I am always surprised at her tremendous strength when she was having her seizure. Even to take a glass out of her hand is next to impossible to pry from her.

I admire her courage and spirit.

Seizure Descriptions

29a

Father Here are a few thoughts and observations from witnessing my daughter have a seizure. First there is no warning as such, maybe a blank stare. If standing, she has always fallen backward, and has hit her head many times on a table, sink, refrigerator, stove and many other objects. She is unconscious during the seizure, her arms and legs shake and sometimes she has some frothing at the mouth. This situation lasts for a few minutes, then she will regain consciousness and be very tired, and sleep a half hour or more. She had a seizure walking across the street one day, fell and broke her jaw. Many, many times she has hit her head with tremendous force.

My thoughts are that some of these seizures are possibly brought on by "state of mind." She looks back at life and considers how things should have been and dwells on the past. Keeping busy and looking ahead seems to help her. From what she tells me her seizures are under control to a greater extent now than ever before. Maybe it is the right combination of medication, or age might have a bearing.

She has had a rough life. Let's hope a cure can be found for epilepsy.

29b

Friend My husband and I have seen our friend go into a seizure only 2 or 3 times. She would start with her hands shaking violently, then she would fall back. We'd put her on her side and she would shake violently all over for about 10 or 15 minutes. She would have no control over her bowels and urine. When she'd come out of it she'd be in a fog for another 10 or 20 minutes. She would then be so tired.

30

Mother Before my daughter has a seizure she is talking to me normally and then her head twitches 3 times to the side and she has a staring look. It lasts seconds and she resumes her conversation (mostly by repeating what I had just said or something she just said). She doesn't seem to know that she just lost seconds but does feel her head twitching. To my knowledge, before she was medicated, I am the only member of the family to have seen the seizure. Also, if you were not looking at her, you wouldn't be aware it was happening.

The first time I saw her have a seizure I was alarmed that something was wrong but I didn't panic.

31a

Friend One day, as my friend and I were about to go to a funeral, I was about to get into her car (in the front) when my friend all of a sudden gave this blank stare and proceeded to slump on the pavement. I tried to grab her, but couldn't (yet she still hung on me). Both my assistant and I looked at her. She had a very somber/subdued expression on her face.

After she realized she had hit the pavement, she kept telling us "That was a piece of ice she slipped on." Both my assistant and I knew that there wasn't any ice around her car and that she was denying she had a seizure. All of this happened within 30 seconds. After we finally got her up off the pavement, into the car, did she realize she must have had a seizure.

There have been other times when she has been at my house. She had offered to help with me serving or bringing things in and out of a room. She can be very bubbly one minute and the next minute her personality changes to a somber expression without facial expression. Her hands begin to shake, she begins to lose touch with reality and does not comprehend what is going on. She ends up dropping or spilling things on the floor.

Just recently, she called me after she had a big seizure. She described it to me; the feeling of helplessness and despair. She blamed it on not having breakfast. Luckily, she was able to get herself off the floor and onto a couch. Her voice was extremely shaky.

There have been many times where she and I will be having a conversation and all of a sudden, she pauses, hesitates, and stops in the middle of a sentence, gets very confused about what we were talking about. She can't comprehend the whole conversation we had just had. To me, this is a clear indication that she had just had another seizure.

I have seen this time after time with her. She tries so hard to be a "normal person" and hide the fact that she has epilepsy. She constantly denies the fact that she has had a seizure. It isn't until I take her step by step from beginning to end (of her seizure) that she realizes that she really did have a seizure.

I have gone over and over with her that it is vitally important for her to ask for help. She needs to let people know she is feeling uneasy and most important be very open and to communicate with her husband.

31b

Husband Having been married to my wife for over seventeen years, I have witnessed many of her seizures. When she has mild seizures and is talking she will usually stop in mid-sentence, stare straight ahead and then start speaking again where she originally left off. If walking, the pace slows down, then speeds back up again. When eating, her right arm shakes. She has several of these seizures a day.

Occasionally, she has big seizures. I have not witnessed many of these. She has usually had these during the day (when I am at work) or in bed at night. They usually start with mild shaking (either arm or leg). Shortly after that, her arms, legs and head shake. During the seizure I make sure there are no objects around that can injure her. I just let the seizure take its course. She usually wants to go to bed and rest after a seizure, so I just let her sleep.

I witnessed my first seizure prior to our marriage. She was careful to let me know about her epilepsy and what to do. I was generally aware of what to expect, but did not realize the shaking would last as long. I had a better understanding of the need for sleep/rest needed due to the energy the body must utilize during a seizure and the unconsciousness and disorientation resulting from it.

31c

Friend I witnessed my friend having seizures one morning at my home. She had slept over the night before. I heard a loud bang coming from upstairs. I went up to see if she was alright. She was sitting on the bathroom floor. I managed to get her onto the bed. She laid on the bed and periodically, but close together, her leg started jerking. At times her whole body would jerk and her jaw would open and close. It mainly was her legs and arms. But this was, maybe, every 30 seconds or so. I'm not sure how long it lasted. After about 5 minutes I told her to lie still and I went downstairs to leave her alone. Maybe 30 minutes later she came downstairs and as she was standing she fell over. It seemed like her knees buckled from under her. Then she seemed fine after that.

32a

Mother Right before a seizure her eyes open very wide and she stares. If we are in a conversation it's apparent that she's trying to concentrate, but her concentration is interrupted. She sometimes moves her head all around and sometimes her hands. Or she might clear her throat a couple of times.

After a seizure she might say "what" a few times and walk around. She comes right back to normal right away.

32b

Sister She is my sister and I have seen her have a number of seizures. She seems to go into a blank stare and it seems like her mouth gets very dry. I will try to talk to her to help her come out of it. When she starts to come out of it, she doesn't really know what's going on. She will say something like "I think I'm supposed to go somewhere tonight, but I can't remember."

She will gradually start to come around and know what's going on. When she has a seizure at home, she will always call either my sister, my brother or me. I can always tell when she's had a seizure just by talking to her on the phone. She will say "Hi" real quick and ask me what I'm doing. After a couple of minutes she knows what is going on.

33

Mother The first time my son had a big seizure was a very frightening time to me because I did not know what was happening to him. He was about seven years old and we were with friends just arriving home from lunch (pizza) out. He became unresponsive and sort of in a frozen state in the car and began turning very blue and then almost black and I picked him up and rushed him into the house, carrying him, and someone called the police for help. As he lay on a couch it seemed we were "losing" him as he did not seem to be breathing—then his arms, legs and body began to jerk in erratic motions. It was very, very frightening and I know I was panic-stricken. He was rushed to the hospital in a police cruiser, with the officer telling me to breathe into his mouth. There was no warning this was going to happen.

Time and years have passed and we have had many of these episodes, usually without warnings, but sometimes he calls out "Help" and repeats "I'll be alright," and then becomes very red in the face, eyes clutched and passes out with some jerking motions of the extremities. The jerking then seems to be only on his left side. We do call for an ambulance and have him checked out at the hospital. He comes around slowly with color coming back in his face and he is exhausted, emotionally upset and has a headache.

It is always a scary time for me, but I know now what to expect and try for his sake to be calm and assure him he is O.K. I know he is the one who must live with this. With the knowledge and understanding now after all these years, I believe it is easier for me.

Seizure Descriptions

I am totally, completely grateful to those doctors and researchers who have dedicated their lives to helping people like my son, who must endure this overwhelming disease. He has come a long way, thanks to his doctors, and lives a pretty good life.

34a

Friend She is my best friend. We met twelve years ago when we both started our new jobs. By the time I first witnessed her seizures I knew her for about a year. I still vividly remember the whole scene.

We just came out from a train station. My friend had to pick up her car after repair and I was heading home. We were talking and suddenly she started to look and act quite strange: her eyes became wide open, yet she did not see anything. She was walking straight ahead and became less and less alert and assertive. She looked completely withdrawn, with no sense of where she was or where she was going to. She did not hear anything and did not respond to any of my questions at all. She looked like she was "far away" mentally and was present there just physically.

First, I thought she was joking or pretending, but then I did not know what to think at all. I just knew that something was very wrong with her. It was all happening so suddenly. I started to consider immediate medical help.

Gradually she started "coming back." It took about ten minutes from the beginning to her first questions: "Where am I? What street it is? What town?" She fully recovered from this seizure in about five minutes and became her normal self again.

I witnessed more of her seizures but usually they were shorter and her recovery was also faster. She knew almost instantly where she was and what was going on around her. *15*

Mother My daughter never appeared to have an aura before her seizures. We could be writing, sewing or dressing the baby. She would just stop doing whatever and stare into space or at me. During a seizure she was usually speechless and always motionless. There seemed to be no eye movement. At times she might speak but lose her trend of thought. Almost as quickly as the seizure came on she would "awaken." I don't recall whether she was ever able to continue our conversation without a reminder of the topic. However if she was doing something, she was able to just continue whatever she was doing.

As time went by, it was obvious they were not only more frequent but were lasting much longer. One particular time we were taking a walk. She just stopped for a few moments and suddenly continued to walk as if nothing had happened. At another time she started talking about our state. I tried to carry this conversation but was unable to. She couldn't answer my questions (as if she didn't hear them) and just continued to talk. After the seizure I questioned her about the conversation and she was unable to recollect any of it. Finally when I realized I was unable to reach her, I just waited until her seizure was over and then would continue whatever we were doing.

How helpless I felt! What can I do? Who do we turn to for help? I am unable to put into words my concern for her, her husband and child. This is my daughter. Here is this young, vivacious, independent (so independent) person unable to live a full life. Is she going to get better or worse? What does the future hold? The only thing to do is get the best medical help and continue with living.

Speaking for myself, her father, siblings and the entire family, we are forever grateful for the concern given her. Since her surgery

Seizure Descriptions

for the seizures, she's her "old self" again and we are most happy
for that.   *15*

35

Son My father sometimes gets seizures when he is standing or
sitting. When he is standing his hands get stiff and he drools. He
also falls or lays down. When his hands are stiff and he drools, his
eyes don't blink and sometimes he says words that we don't know in
our language. When he is sitting down he does the same things but
he puts his head down.

36

Husband My spouse has three different types of seizures. Before all
of the seizures she has an aura. Sometimes during the aura she will
just have a blank stare on her face and then it passes quickly, but
mostly she will say that she is going down and that she is sorry that
she is having the seizure because it is ruining my life. This upsets
me. She shouldn't be sorry that she has seizures because she does
her best to control them, and because they aren't ruining my life and
she shouldn't feel that way.

As for the seizure, if it turns out to be just an aura, it stops at this
point and she is okay. If it turns out to be a blackout, she may do
many different things. She may just sit and stare blankly, she may
have a twitch in one of her eyes, she may grab objects such as pencils
and play with them, she may kick her legs in bicycle like manner,
and she may wet herself. One really doesn't know what she is going

to do when she goes into one—it is totally unpredictable. If it is a big one it will usually come if she has already had a blackout during the day, but this may not always be true. During a big one she will go into convulsions in which her whole body will shake. Often it may be only one side, such as the left eye twitching and the left leg shaking. She will usually make grunting sounds and breathe quite heavily. It is impossible to control her and you just have to hope that she won't hurt herself.

Typically, I am a little scared when a seizure starts. After that, I sort of have to almost distance myself from the fact that this is my wife and just begin to time how long the seizure lasts. Also, I have to make sure that nothing is around that can hurt her, such as sharp objects or scissors, and that she won't strike her head. When she has come out of the seizure, I have to ask her if she knows where she is, what day it is, and questions of that nature until she knows what is going on. It will usually take her 15–30 seconds before she becomes familiar with her surroundings. If she is having a convulsion I try to wait for her to come out of it, but occasionally I have to call the ambulance.

Afterwards, if it was an aura, she will be fine, with no problems. If it was a blackout she may look weary and tired. It will usually take a little bit of time (30 seconds–1 minute) before color comes back to her cheeks. She will often look fine fairly quickly and be able to go back to what she was doing. Occasionally, she will look very pale and haggard, and be quite limp (as though her body is just dead weight). She then usually will go straight to bed. If it was a convulsion, all she can do is sleep it off. She will go into a deep sleep that is hard to rouse her from. But once she has slept it off, she will be okay.

The first time I saw my wife have a seizure I felt a little nervous. We were on a bus so I sort of looked around to see if other passengers noticed, but they didn't seem to. I knew she had epilepsy, so

Seizure Descriptions

I was prepared for it, but I didn't really know what to think. I really was just concerned for her safety, and I guess I felt sort of sorry for her that she had to go through this experience.

37

Wife When I first saw my husband take a seizure, I was talking to him and he did not answer me back. He stared and did not respond.

Usually, he makes a noise with his lips. He has a taste in his mouth and smacks his lips. He has very small seizures. If he misses 1–2 doses of pills he usually has a small seizure the next day. He gets very tired after a seizure and says to me he feels all alone with no one around.

If he is under a lot of pressure or something bothers him it may bring a seizure on. I will say, you just had a seizure. He said he did not.

38a

Co-worker I can't exactly remember the first time I saw my co-worker have one because it was a long while ago. The first time though, I was kind of shocked, because you'll be having a conversation with her and she just blanks out likes she's lost. She doesn't understand you and she doesn't even know where she is or who she is. I found it to be strange and a little scary. They usually last between 3 to 5 minutes. When she starts to come out of the seizure, she's kind of spaced out and tired and drawn looking. You really can't say what happens before a seizure, because it always happens so fast. One minute she is talking to a customer or cashing out a check, and all of a sudden she spaces out, stands in one place and stares. I ask her questions like, "Where are you?" and she looks at you like you're talking in a foreign language; she stays dazed for awhile after the seizure. *11*

38b

Daughter My mother has had seizures since the eighth month she was pregnant with me, so most of it I don't remember.

I guess the earliest memory I have is when she taught me to drive a car at age twelve in case she had a seizure. At that time, she knew when she was having one, so she would tell me and then either pull over or ask for help. The early ones lasted 2–3 minutes and then she was fine, and the day went on.

The next vivid memory was when I was about fifteen years old. I was at a skating rink waiting for her to pick me up and waited and waited. The police showed up and told me my mother had a seizure and drove the wrong way through an intersection and didn't remember anything; I guess that was the changing point to the seizures. She stopped driving a car, and her seizures have generally stayed the same since. From then on, she would not know when she was having one.

When I was young, I guess I could have fun with her when she had one by asking questions she couldn't answer like: "Who am I?" or "Where are you?"

To me, they are a part of my life and normal activity to take care of them. So sometimes I dismiss it as "no big deal." But I guess it must be a big deal to her. *11*

Seizure Descriptions

Fiancé The first time my fiancée had a seizure in my presence was a couple of months ago. We were having lunch with two friends, a gentleman and his wife. Although she (who is always up front) told me about her epilepsy, I did not know what to expect. Had she not told me, when it happened my first thought would be to get medical attention immediately. Having been told, I just sat and wondered how can I help this woman? No resolution.

She seemed to be unconscious; her eyes were blank, her face appeared soft and relaxed. I knew she was alive, but her mental functions seemed to have stopped. In perhaps an interval of two minutes, she seemed to wake up and asked, "What's going on?"

By now I have seen her experience a number of seizures. Looking back to before the seizure, she and I had been discussing something, or I was attempting to explain something to her, or she herself was attempting to tell me something, and her mental functions just stopped, and that's the seizure.

Now that I have seen her have several seizures, it seems like her brain is the center of a communications system where all information is sent to this center and when its capacity has been reached, everything just stops. *11*

39

Mother My son has taken seizures since he was 2½ years old. He has been hospitalized and has taken every different pill on the market and nothing has helped.

When he has a seizure there is no warning. He just stops whatever he is doing and makes funny sounds and walks around. His right hand and arm seem to stiffen up and sometimes tremble and sometimes he stares off into space and seems to lean to the right as if to fall but he doesn't fall. He is in this position about two to three minutes, then he will wander around as if he is looking for something. After about 2 to 3 seconds of this he takes off his clothes and looks for his pajamas. He is still very incoherent and without a clue to where he is. After about 5 minutes he comes out of it and proceeds to do what he was doing before he had the seizure. Other times he may just lie down and fall asleep for a few minutes.

If he has a seizure when he is lying or sitting down he will just stare off into space with his right hand moving on its own. He also at times clicks his teeth or chews. These usually last 2 to 3 minutes. The seizure is then followed by a period of confusion lasting from 3 to 5 minutes during which he might undress. If he's home he'll change into his pajamas and go to bed and fall asleep for about 5 to 20 minutes. Other times he will look for something but he doesn't know what, or he will put the bread into his socks, or have trouble performing simple functions such as shutting off the television. He can also be very hard to reason with at this time. But once he regains his senses he is back to normal.

40a

Co-worker About a year and a half ago, two women I work with brought to my attention that our friend was totally ignoring them. (The three women work together in the same cubicle.) They complained that on several occasions when they spoke to her, she would ignore them. Once I went to their cubicle to pick up some work and one of them said, "I don't know what's wrong—but she is totally ignoring us." When I went over to look at her, she was gazing into her computer screen. I called her name and she didn't respond. I looked at the other two women and said "wait a minute." I went back to my desk and called her on the phone. After about two rings she answered the phone in a normal manner! When she was away from her desk I asked the other two how often this happened. They said about three or four times this past week. I looked at one of them and asked her when she was going to talk to our co-worker's father again. I said that I thought she could be having seizures. I had a good friend in school that had seizures and I read up on them and suggested that we call our friend's father and let him know. That's when she went to the doctors and found out that's what was actually happening to her. At first we all thought maybe she was distracted by her wedding plans and her grandmother's illness, but when she started having five or six a day we became deeply concerned. We were heartbroken when we found out what was actually wrong.

40b

Husband My wife first experienced seizure activity nearly two years ago. We were planning our wedding at that time and the date was about eight months away. Our family, friends and co-workers believed the seizure was from wedding jitters and excitement.

Now, she averages twelve to fifteen seizures per month. Strangely her seizures seem to cluster together. She can go one and one half weeks without having a seizure and the following three to seven days she can have two, three, even six a day.

When a seizure occurs it's like she's daydreaming or spacing out. She asks what time is it and what day is it. She does pretty much everything normally; subconsciously she's fine. Some examples are taking a shower, getting into a car or giving me a smile, hug and a kiss. She doesn't get an aura before a seizure occurs. There is no warning.

The last seizure she had was last Father's day. The phase after the seizure lasted about three hours. That morning she felt shaky and tired. She was spaced out and daydreaming. She tried walking upstairs at a restaurant and her legs buckled under her and she fell to the ground. I was by her side and she did not get hurt. She said "help me, help me," as if she knew something was wrong. Most of all she was extremely confused and did not know where she was. Eventually she came out of it and she was fine. She had two other similar experiences to date. Her legs were weak and that is what caused her to buckle like that. I pray she never has to go through this again.

This whole situation is hard to accept. After all, we are newly-weds. Our wedding was a year ago. It is a big adjustment getting used to each other and so on. No one wants to see a loved one go through this. One thing that has helped me is having such a wonderful wife. I'm in the medical field as an x-ray tech. That gives me some understanding. I'm exposed to so many things in my field. I had only seen one type of seizure—convulsive seizures. I came to learn that there are many types of seizures and that they affect people in many different ways. Sometimes I feel so helpless because I can't take away the pain she goes through dealing with her seizures. I wish I could make them go away.

I am very supportive of my wife and try my best to keep her in good spirits as much as I can. I tell her this whole situation could be much worse, so let's be thankful. I do not want my wife going through this for the rest of her life. I pray this can be controlled through medication and that this nightmare will be over.

Seizure Descriptions

This has affected our lives. Ever since her first seizure we ask ourselves, why is this happening? We learned to accept it and deal with it the best we can and the possibility that this might never go away. She does not drive a car either. She rarely goes anywhere by herself. In a way she's afraid to.

It's a big change in her life because she just cannot get up and go out on her own and drive to the store. She loses her independence. She depends on others to take her places. I take her wherever she wants to go, as do our family and friends. Everyone gives her all the support that she needs.

In closing, I learnt a great deal from this situation. Never take life and good health for granted. Life is too short. Life could be a lot worse so let's be grateful and appreciate what we have and thank the Lord. I hope and pray there will be some type of cure for this disorder.

40c

Mother-in-law The first time I saw my daughter-in-law have a seizure, she was at my home and she got very confused as to where she was and what she had in her pocketbook. She was looking at papers but had no idea as to what they were. It only lasted a few minutes and after it was over, she was fine.

As time went by and she had other seizures, I would notice different things, like her speech would not make sense and her eyes would get glassy. She was never violent or loud and she never used any bad language.

The only thing that worries and scares me is if she ever had a seizure when she was alone outside or taking public transportation by herself. Her seizures only last a few minutes and a few have lasted longer but in those few minutes something could happen.

41a

Mother-in-law When I heard the word, epilepsy, sheer dread went through me. This only happened to other families, other people. This is a condition that dates back to Biblical times; known as "Holy Man disease." Why should this be thrust upon my son-in-law? What will my daughter have to bear? How will this affect my 2 grand-daughters? Will their lifestyle be forever changed? In total panic I called my doctor and asked if he could set aside time for me as I needed to talk to him and get all the information possible. He was most kind and I spent an hour with him, after his normal office hours. When I returned home I was still very upset. Only once have I wit-nessed someone having a seizure—many years ago—and the sight of it came back to me—and it wasn't pretty.

I asked my daughter whether her 2 girls had seen their father during a seizure and if they did, what their reaction was. For many nights after, I could not sleep. My days were filled with my job, but every free moment my thoughts were with my son-in-law and my daughter and how they were coping. I went to the library and read whatever I could on epilepsy. I called the local epilepsy foundation and got several leaflets from them.

Instead of calling them once a week, as usual, my calls went up to 3 or 4 times a week, until my daughter told me to please go back to the normal once a week. I did as she asked and then realized that repeating the same thing so many times may only do damage to them. My life was in a turmoil just waiting to hear, week by week,

Seizure Descriptions

how he was doing and perhaps I felt some guilt because I couldn't be with them, even if it was only for moral support. My job kept me away but I assured both of them that I would come up to them, no matter what, if they needed me.

Right now I do see a change in him for the better. Of course, I fully realize that he still has a long, hard road ahead. Both my son-in-law and daughter are fully confident that it may take a while. There may be a setback once in a while, but not doing anything would be worse. With the advances the medical field has made, I'm sure that shortly a cure will be found.

41b

Wife So much denial, so much pain and frustration. Blaming anything and everything except the fact that my husband has epilepsy! Not understanding what is going on and worrying every time he is 5 minutes late getting home from work. I tell the children, "Don't bother Daddy . . . don't trouble him with your problems." Afraid that if he gets upset and has a disagreement with any of us . . . will it cause another seizure? Is there something in the carpet so he can't stay with me in our own family room? Is it the house? Maybe we should put the house on the market. Even blaming it on the air quality. Would a job in another state be better? Be different?

We limit the amount of friends we have. Are we shutting the world out or closing ourselves in? At the beginning, he had 1–2 seizures a year. We're told it's allergy related. One day, I call the house and find out my husband of a year or so was rushed to the hospital. I come home and find him on his back. Two vertebrae in his back are broken from falling off a chair. How the chair fell, I don't know. All I know was that the paramedics lifted him incorrectly.

Being very young and naive, I did not comprehend what was going on and didn't understand why my husband is going to a neurologist.

Years go by and nothing occurs. All I know is every so often he tells me about "funny feelings" going on in his head.

A series of tests are performed at a hospital. Trying to bring on a seizure. He is exposed to everything and anything but to everyone's dismay, nothing. However, physicians labeled what we both thought from the beginning. Epilepsy.

I felt a sigh of relief and a haunting fear. What does this entail? A friend of ours tells me of a neurologist at another hospital, when we're ready. The physician locally could only do so much. Perhaps there is a future for all of us. We speak to the neurologist and tell him all that has happened. Gradually, my husband is going through tests, being wired, probed and filmed; and all the while, I'm there— need to be there, but I'm also a mother and have certain responsibilities. Taking over roles, making decisions, being a chauffeur—my husband does not have his license—is all encompassing. When will I get off the treadmill?

After many months of testing and decision making, it was determined brain surgery would be the answer. Our choice? We had none.

The children were being prepared; talking to staff, social workers, people at the hospital extending themselves to them. The waiting was terrifying. I was always filled with doubt, full of what ifs, but slowly worked towards a positive outlook. My husband's parents are told; my mother and 5 of our closest friends are told that he is going in for surgery and everything is explained. They say laughter is the best medicine. I must have been hysterical! The day of surgery comes, and the phone rings at 6 in the morning. It's my husband telling me how they came in and prepped him and how they were to shave his head, sounding as if he were a lamb being led to slaughter. I try to reassure him, saying I wouldn't stand for anything else but 100%.

Seizure Descriptions

It is now a little over 3 years, and we are trying to get our lives and ourselves back together. We're re-establishing our life and taking it one day at a time!

41c

Daughter The fact that my father had epilepsy never really ffected me much, rather I should say that I did not allow it to affect me. I had too many things on my mind to sit and sulk over it. I have always felt that what happens, happens, and there is not much that you can do to change that. When I first found out about my father's epilepsy I was a freshman in high school.

It was right before Thanksgiving break and we were getting ready to go on a trip. I came home early and everything appeared to be fine. Things can often change in a split second though. The next thing, I realized, was that my father was acting very strange and having a seizure. At the time I had no idea what was going on, because my parents thought that at the time I really didn't need to know. I called my mom at work and she rushed right home. Later that day they explained everything to me and then it was my turn to explain everything to my sister. During the continuation of my father's epilepsy this is how things usually went. My dad would have a seizure, doors would close, and then if anything needed to be done it was up to me. When it came to chores and household things, I became the mother, replacing my mother while she was with my father in the hospital. During my freshman year in college my father went in for his operation. I had to keep everything together, not just for me, but for the rest of my family. When my grandparents needed their fears calmed, I was the one who did it. When my sister needed reassuring, I was the one who did it. The roles were completely reversed: I was the mother and even if at times I did not want the job, I was stuck with it.

Little by little things did improve though. When my dad came home from the hospital both my parents, I think, tried very hard to make things about as normal as things could be. With the financial troubles and other backlashes of his epilepsy, things really couldn't be that normal. Everyday we seemed to be reminded that we were not a typical normal family, but one of us had a problem that affected all of us. I wouldn't say that I am regretful about anything that has happened to me or my family as a whole. The events have made me a stronger, much more independent person than I think my parents appreciated at times.

Overall I would say to families that are going through the same thing that you should not try to deal with all of the problems by yourselves. At times, I admit, I felt left out as if the only thing that did matter was my father and everything else came a distant second. Many events were cut short, or in cases even dismissed and that did bother me, but in the long run you get used to it and realize that there are other things that are important.

41d

Daughter I can't remember a time when it really started. Every once in a while my parents' bedroom door would close and lock and my father wouldn't come out for a long time. Nothing seemed strange to me, since it had always been happening. But then these "every once in a whiles" started to happen more often. Being older, I remember hearing the noises, my mother crying, my father scream-ing. I would go in my room and pretend not to hear. My parents soon realized that matters were getting worse, and that they had to

Seizure Descriptions

give an explanation for these occurrences. I was thirteen years old, on a visit to my grandparents, when I was told that my father had epilepsy, but I didn't know at that time what epilepsy was, or what it had to do with me. When we got home, no one talked about what had been disclosed, and I couldn't seem to get the courage to bring it up. I was scared to be left home alone with him, not knowing what a seizure was or what to do for someone experiencing one. All I knew was that I had to avoid him as much as possible so I wouldn't have to deal with the problem.

I was lucky, since I never actually saw my father having a full blown convulsive seizure, but I did witness him having mild seizures, and saw him in the hospital many times after he had been taken there for treatment. One Sunday morning, though, he survived a double, possibly triple seizure. An ambulance arrived, police cars filled my driveway, and the stretcher was brought into the house and the men attempted to tie my father down to it. Full of fear, not knowing what was happening to him, my father fought back, screaming out my sister's name. My sister and I were told to remain in our rooms, crying, helpless, not knowing what to do. The worst part about this display wasn't having to hear him scream, and it wasn't having to see him in the hospital bed later on, it was having to explain to everyone in my neighborhood what had happened. I was embarrassed by his affliction, I didn't want anyone to know that my family had a problem. For the next few weeks, I made up different stories to tell people.

A little while after the last of three auto accidents, my father's license was taken away by the state. He was told that he was a hazard to other motorists and to himself, like he were some kind of villain. At first I felt so angry that he was being punished for something that he could not prevent, but then I realized that it was probably for the best. My father felt like some kid, chauffeured around by his wife and eldest daughter, not able to go anywhere by himself. He had been so independent, but now, his dignity was gone. He had no privacy and had to rely on others for practically everything.

During the middle of my freshman year, my father switched doctors and hospitals, and things began to move fast. He was sent in for tests to try to isolate the area of his brain that was causing the problem, and after they found it, he was scheduled for brain surgery to remove the faulty region, two weeks into my sophomore year. When I was allowed to see him, the day after his surgery, all I could think about was leaving; it was horrifying. I walked into his room and saw him curled up in the fetal position, his head completely bandaged and his face swollen. He was not able to speak or move. Every day, though, he got a little better. He left the hospital a month later to recover at home and returned to his job a few months after that. Upon returning to work, he anticipated a heartwarming welcome back, but instead, his employers, not believing that he could now do his job better than ever before, cut his salary in half, took away his position and title, and gave him menial tasks to perform. My mother was unemployed and we had a mile high stack of hospital bills to worry about. Before the surgery, we always found a way to make ends meet, but now everything changed, our lifestyles had to be altered to fit our new financial and emotional situation.

During those years, I had mixed feelings for my father. At times I had so much jealousy and rage towards him. He was the center of everyone's world, everything was done for him. I always had to hear about how he felt, but no one ever wanted to know how I felt. I had to suppress my emotions, for fear that they might upset him and instead act like nothing mattered. I built up a wall around myself, so that nothing could hurt me, and now, two years, after the fact, I still have trouble expressing my feelings and the wall hasn't completely fallen down—I can't get over what has happened. I didn't have my mother's attention because of him, I couldn't have nice things

Seizure Descriptions

because of him, I couldn't invite my friends over because of him, I had no free time because of him, I didn't have a father because of him.

I knew these things weren't his fault, but I didn't know who else to blame for shattering my family and my life. At other times, though, I couldn't have loved him more. With every seizure, every car accident, and every hospital visit came the possibility of losing him. I wanted so badly to be close to him but he was so far out of reach. I didn't think that I could talk to him or ask him for anything. My thoughts and concern went to him, to make him better, to end the madness we had to live in.

From the moment my mother told me that my father had epilepsy my life changed. I had to grow up and accept the hardships that were yet to come. Without a mother or father around for us, my sister and I raised each other and ourselves from scared children into mature young adults who could deal with the adversity surrounding us. There are events and other things that I've blocked out, that I can't remember. This scares me, knowing that I've only lived for seventeen years and bits and pieces of two of those years have been erased. I find myself never wanting to sit still. I lost too much time and I need to get it back. I'm not going to say that I am happy about this ordeal, but I am happy about what I learned from it. I realize that the little things aren't that important, only the people you love. I'm more independent and can stand up under some of the most intense pressure. Schoolwork and problems with my friends are nothing compared with what I have had to experience in the past.

The story does have a happy ending though. My father, after a lot of fighting with the legal system, obtained a settlement from his company for their discriminatory actions, and got his license back after being seizure free for over six months. Since that last seizure about two years ago, he hasn't experienced another. The money problems still exist but our lives have been slowly put back together.

Epilepsy in Our View

78

My sister is a junior in college, my mother is employed and my father is more fit and healthy than ever before. He does everything and anything he wants, and I now have a relationship with him that never existed before. I admire him more than anyone else in this world. I could never have survived through what he has. My father, mother, sister and I still have the scars from our experiences, but at least the wounds are healing.

42

Wife The first time I saw my husband have a seizure was 18 years ago. I can remember it like it was yesterday. I had no idea and neither did he that he had epilepsy. I awoke with him thrashing next to me in his sleep. I tried talking to him and was getting no response. His eyes were open and his whole right side was shaking. I called an ambulance. By the time we got him to the hospital he seemed to be fine. The doctors could not tell me what the problem was. About a month after this the same thing occurred, again in an ambulance. We were told at the hospital from the doctor on call that everything seemed to be fine. (Because by the time we got to the hospital he was out of the seizure.) Finally, the third time the doctor on call looked in his eyes (they were dilated) and told me this man just had a seizure. I stood in disbelief! What causes seizures? How long has he had them? Will he be alright? Can he go home and not have another one? So many questions. . . . Where are the answers? The doctor on call told me to make an appointment with a neurologist—he will be able to answer my questions.

His seizures will start at 2 or 3 in the morning. I will be awake until the last one has subsided which could be until 3 or 4 in the morning. He will go back to sleep but be unable to go to work the next day. Depression will set in. I will go to work and come home to find him still in bed. The battle begins—I will argue to get him to get out of bed—tell him to stop feeling sorry for himself—while he says he has no control over how he feels. And he cannot help feeling depressed. How could I understand? I don't have seizures!

43a

Daughter When I see my father have a seizure I feel afraid and nervous. He sometimes stares and sometimes jerks around and bites his tongue. I get very scared because I don't know what will happen next.

My father had a brain operation and since then hasn't had a seizure. I did a science project on seizures and learned a lot about it so now I'm not as scared.   7

43b

Wife When my husband has a seizure, he generally stares. He can stay like this for as little as a minute or as long as two to three hours. He is usually unresponsive, although there are times when he may answer you, but without making sense. He usually has a headache and feels very tired afterwards.

When he has a mild seizure, unless you are aware of them, you most likely will miss it or misinterpret it as someone stopping to collect his thoughts.

A convulsion is the worst. Luckily these did not happen too often. However, when they did the first sign for him would be twitching of his mouth, which was followed immediately by his body thrashing about. The few that I witnessed lasted about 1 to 2 minutes and usually left him with a headache and feeling tired and sore.

The first time he had a convulsion, I wasn't scared until after it was over, than I realized what could have happened—a few minutes more he would have been in the car driving—a few minutes earlier he was holding our 9-month-old daughter. In a way I felt lucky, for all of us, that the seizure happened in the house. I somehow knew that he was okay even though the ambulance took him to the hospital.   7

44

Mother It was a typical summer Sunday, so we decided to take a family drive. We had driven a short distance, when my 6-year-old daughter said, "It smells bad." As I turned to ask her what smelled bad, she repeated, "It smells bad." When my gaze met her face, her eyes were staring in a fixed position to the left. No one else could detect the odor she had sensed.

We immediately started for home. On the return trip (approximately a 10-minute ride) she sat very still. Her eyes remained fixed. She did not respond to any verbal communication.

Upon arrival at home, she was carried to the house. As she was laid on the bed, a slight tensing and twitching motion on the left side of her body was visible. This quickly turned into strong convulsing movements. It was somewhat frightening to witness, as you feel very helpless.

After the convulsing stopped, her body appeared to relax and she slept for a short period of time. As she awoke, she seemed disoriented. She said, "My head hurts." Her father recognized the convulsing, as he was familiar with a similar condition in another family member.

This experience led to visits with doctors and hospitals, and tests. Doctors diagnosed her as having epilepsy. My first reaction to the diagnosis was of mixed emotions. Three, that I recall; Anger . . . that this had to happen to my daughter. Frustration . . . that I could not change it. Sadness . . . that this little girl would have to bear this through her lifetime. As the doctors explained seizure activity (and that it could be controlled by medication) my frustration turned to determination. Determination that my child would not be treated differently than other children. Instead of living in fear of when the next seizure would occur, I realized that epilepsy does not have to control a person's life.

Twenty-four years later, this little 6-year-old girl is now a adult. She has her own apartment to maintain. She carries out her every-day chores and responsibilities . . . with an occasional time-out for seizures.   *6*

45a

Friend I had known my friend for many years before I learned she had seizures. Even after I heard that her seizures were seriously affecting her life, it was several years before I was with her face to face when a seizure occurred.

She and I were going shopping together and she let me know that she had been having many seizures that day. She told me what to expect and how to help. Initially I was terrified, feeling an awe-some responsibility for her safety. Just as she predicted, a seizure came on with a soft crying sound and I put my arm around her to keep her from falling, as she had instructed. During her seizure, she looked very sad and continued to make sounds as if she were crying. It passed quickly and after a moment, she regained her thought process and we continued on. Other times there seems to be "after shocks" that keep her from renewing her thoughts and conversation for several minutes.

Once, when I wasn't aware of any warning sounds, she fell and I was astounded by the suddenness. I don't remember any of the convulsive movements I had been prepared to expect. She continued her crying sounds for several seconds and then became aware of having fallen. As I knew how upsetting it was for her to get attention from strangers, I let everyone know she was fine and we moved on. When she had seizures during our lunches together, I was initially afraid she would choke on her food but I was relieved to see that this never seemed to be a problem. I remember feeling grateful that we were sitting down and so she couldn't fall.

As we have gone out together over the past few years, I have become less apprehensive and more confident that I can be helpful if a seizure occurs. I feel strongly that my ability to relax with her is directly related to her attitude that she is prepared to go on with as normal a life as possible and deal with the negative results of a seizure if she has to. Her directness in preparing me for what may happen that particular day and her ability to make me feel that she, not I, is responsible for her well-being has made it much less stressful to be together. In fact, we have fun together!

45b

Friend I don't remember when precisely I first encountered one of my friend's seizures. I knew (she had probably told me) that she had a continuing "condition." We were part of an ongoing poetry workshop, and her poems often dealt with the experience of someone having a seizure. For a very long time, I had known her in many ways; poet, single mother, social worker, and friend. None of these had anything to do with her being a "seizure victim." I remember once talking with her on the phone, and having her simply disappear. And once talking with her at a party, the same thing happened. But in neither case were there any visible, physical signs of her condition. Then again, I really had no idea what the signs would be. My only prior experience with seizures was with a substitute teacher in junior high school who was rumored (with extravagant, embroidered detail, of course) to "fall into a fit" if the class was too unruly. None of us was ever brave or foolish enough to put that to the test.

One day we were having lunch. All of a sudden, and at a moment when the conversation was not a bit humorous, she seemed to be overtaken by a fit of giggling. Her face turned red, her whole body shook, and she made an odd, gentle, persistent sound, rather like someone laughing at the wrong moment, and trying to conceal it. Or she might have been crying, I suppose.

In any case, it took some time for it to dawn on me what was happening. She apologized when the seizure was over (she always does, as if it were somehow irresponsible of her to have the seizures). That reaction puzzled me, but now makes total sense, since I've had my own bout with a neurological "anomaly," as the doctors like to call it. It is a total loss of control, and it feels shameful and guilt-inducing.

It was much later that I witnessed, in a manner of speaking, one of the falls which often accompany her seizures. We were all at a party, in the home of one of our poet friends. Much of the party seemed to have migrated to the kitchen, perhaps because it was the one room in the house not full of breakable nick-knacks, the one room where someone as large and clumsy as I am could feel at ease. Suddenly there was the sound of a breaking glass and a dreadful *thump*, followed by a scurry of activity with my friend (prone on the floor) in the middle. Someone carefully picked up the broken shards of the glass of seltzer she had dropped, someone else took her arm as she got up, and walked upstairs with her to a spare bedroom, where she could lie down and rest.

I've encountered her falls a few times since. When we walk on the street, I nervously hold her arm, as if I could prevent her falling to the pavement. When we have lunch together, and head home in different ways on the subway, I always leave a little guiltily, sure she will fall as soon as I'm out of sight and earshot, as in fact she has, occasionally.

I ponder her life a good deal, not just because we are good friends. She of course doesn't drive a car, which is a major problem. But she works (in the adoption system when I first knew her; now, as a trained social worker, running groups for seizure sufferers and their families), and functions as a single parent of two children. She writes (although she has recently taken a prolonged sabbatical from writing; just because, in a situation well-known to all of us who write, "the poems just won't come").

I've told her, more than once—she hates for me to say it, but it's true—that she is, to me, a kind of hero or role model, in maintaining a largely "normal" life in spite of a potentially incapacitating condition. I look at her with something approaching—yes, it's the right word for it—awe, since I'm fully aware that I couldn't do it, and might conceivably have to. Another friend of mine, who is visually impaired, is quite angry about our tendency to see "heroism" in the living of a normal life with the added limitation of what is crudely called a "disability." I suppose that is what I am doing in claiming a kind of heroism for her. But I know, from my own long bout of rehabilitation, how much energy and tactical thinking is involved in her life, and how deftly and readily she manages it. If the word "heroism" is too ponderous (and too stereotyping), how about "guts"?

Still, when I am around her I cannot get away from the worry— if she has a seizure, what should I *do*? Make the seizure stop?

Seizure Descriptions

85

Hardly—even high-powered neurologists don't seem up to that task. Make the seizures go away? Short of some sort of mystical healing power, that doesn't seem very likely either. Pretend it just isn't happening? But that's an insult to her intelligence, after all. Maybe what I can do is avoid the impulse to hover and—aside from getting some sort of medical attention, if her fall has done something like open a gash on her forehead—help her deal with the embarrassment and shame. Refuse to acknowledge there is any need or justification for apology. Pick up the conversation (with maybe a small recapitulation) and move on. Do, in short, what she does—live, with a considerable but not in the end "crippling" difficulty. Live a full, intelligent, humane and thoughtful life. Be a friend but not a surrogate parent. Offer a hand if she asks for it, but just keep on truckin', as the old song puts it. And never forget: she's a person, and a remarkably talented one, too, not a "victim" or a "cripple" and certainly not an object of pity.

46a

Mother When my son starts to have a seizure, he becomes very still. Then his eyes become unfocused. If he is leaning on the table in front of him his right hand drifts toward the right pushing whatever is in the way with his hand. He seems to be trying to keep himself steady. His right arm rises as if to find balance level. It is then that either his wife or I grab hold on his hand to steady him. I can feel the tension ease in him as he works out of the seizure. It lasts no longer than one minute. After the seizure, he feels discouraged and depressed. There doesn't seem to be any motivation for the seizures. They happen unexpectedly and sometimes in clusters.

When I first saw a seizure I was frightened. I didn't know what was happening. That was a long time ago and I can't say I am any the less apprehensive now.   *5*

46b

Nephew My uncle doesn't often have seizures when I am with him, but when he does, I notice that he looks dazed and pale during the ten to twenty second seizure. Sometimes raises his right arm, though seemingly unaware of the action. If he has a seizure while standing up, he loses his balance and is in danger of falling.   *5*

46c

Sister My brother seems to get a "fixed" look in his eyes when he begins a seizure. He appears to be looking into the middle distance, and then his body often lists a bit to the side. Sometimes he raises his right arm a bit in the course of the 15–20 second seizure, and his hand often shows some sign of tremor. After the seizure is over, he is generally anxious to assure us that he is fine, although it does seem that it takes him a few more minutes to completely regain his composure.   *5*

47a

Case Manager I am writing in response to your request for observations concerning my client's seizure activity. I have been her case manager for about a year. There is no pattern to when seizures happen. It appears to me that she becomes pale at the onset of a seizure. She will begin to drool, her limbs become rigid and she will drop her head and upper body to the left. She has never fallen to my knowledge. As a safety precaution, she sits in an arm chair when at work. I have seen her respond to verbal suggestions to wipe her mouth and hold her head up. This only happens when her seizures have been brief. She has received much attention from peers, who will actually hold her up and express verbal concerns. I have asked that her peers refrain from this and assure them that the staff will assist her. It has been my impression that this attention from peers tends to prolong the after effects of the seizures as she is able to respond to prompts and is smiling.

There have been times when her seizures will continue off and on throughout the morning. During this time she is not able to respond to staff and requires physical assistance to sit in the chair since she tends to slide. It is during these times that I will have her go home. It usually will take two of us to get her into the car.

47b

Father My daughter's seizures take many forms. Sometimes her limbs are stiff, her head turns and her eyes turn inward. She also sweats quite a bit. She is unable to move and has to be carried and put to bed. After a one or two hour nap, she is back to her old self. She is able to respond when you speak to her with a smile or a few words. In another type of seizure, she is functioning normally but her lips and tongue are moving.

Probably the worst type of seizure is one of vomiting. You never know how long it will last. This happens about two or three times a year. There is little stiffness of limbs but she is very tired.

We first noticed her seizures when she was about 6 or 7 months old. She was unable to sit up and her eyes would turn. Naturally it was very traumatic for my wife and me.

47c

Mother When my daughter has a seizure, she has this involuntary motion with her lips and sometimes jerking of her leg. Also, at times her eyes roll and other times she sweats. After the seizures, she needs to sleep one hour and she has weakness in her leg (either left or right). Sometimes she is unable to walk at all and at other times she can with some assistance.

48

Mother My son appears to have two types of seizures. The first type will happen fairly frequently. In the middle of a conversation he will just stop and develop a blank look. This usually lasts about a minute or less and he will continue on with the conversation exactly where he left off.

The bigger seizures usually begin with a period of confusion. He will wander around his room looking for something such as clothing or a book but not find it. Just a quiet state of confusion which can last for half an hour and sometimes longer, ending with falling down and jerking, biting his tongue, having his muscles tighten, jerking some more, perspiring and eventually quieting down and appearing to be asleep. When he comes to, he feels stiff and achy and will sleep for several hours.

Seizure Descriptions

I have noticed that a seizure can follow something stressful happening in his life.

At present he is taking medication which does seem to control the seizures quite well. His convulsions are infrequent—several months to a year apart and have almost always happened shortly after waking up.

As to how I feel viewing a seizure—helpless, scared and upset of course. He usually falls and hurts himself in some way.

49a

Father My daughter's first seizures occurred at the age of 6 when I was away from home. The first direct observation I had was when she was in high school. My wife and I heard her cry out at a nocturnal seizure. Our response was to inform her doctor, and somewhat belatedly support her wish for therapy/counseling. This concern intensified when she reported a seizure at college.

It was much later when I finally saw a seizure. My concern was "what to do" and I was so ill-informed that I tried to put my fingers in her mouth to ensure its openness. Thereafter I observed two drop seizures in the dining room, and about six seizures when driving her.

Looking back, I should have been far more aggressive in consulting the medical practitioners involved, and exploiting the degree of consultation and pooling of information (i.e., x-rays and what happened to them) than I was. Whether or not that would have helped in the critical early years, I don't know.

But I should have tried harder.

Mother My daughter suffers from a seizure disorder which has been through several phases. I was present at the first episode in this disorder and can describe it and my reactions as follows.

She was just short of her sixth birthday. We were in my family's summer house, and we had a young woman from the Netherlands staying with us. Her sister was three and her brother was 15 months old. We had been out for the morning, visiting a local doctor who had prescribed an antibiotic medication for an infection in her ear. We were having lunch outdoors around a picnic table when I noticed that she wasn't with us. She was over by the front steps and looked strange. I remember going over to her and realizing that she was vomiting in a slow, peculiar way. I spoke to her with some urgency and got no response. I sat down on the step and gathered her into my lap. She just sat there, retching slowly and rhythmically, giving no response.

We got her upstairs to a bedroom and took note of the symptoms: eyes open, retching subsided, but no response! Suddenly, I saw the right side of her body give a massive shudder. It was unlike anything else I had ever seen. Then she was still. I called the doctor. He was out. I left a message that it was important to call me right away. Time went by. I called again. Still out! Finally, I got hold of him and held a rather stilted conversation. I must have failed to communicate any urgency (I am a pediatrician's daughter myself and spent a childhood hearing about overanxious mothers.) Suddenly, something I said got the doctor's attention, "You mean she doesn't respond at all?" This was followed by a quick directive to bring her over to his office as fast as possible. Once there, I lifted her onto his table. He tested her reactions with a light needle scratch—first to one foot, then the other. One foot withdrew, the other did not. "I don't like this, I don't like this at all," he muttered. "You'll want to go to the hospital, won't you?" he said.

Now I was traveling with my daughter, our friend and the two younger children. I suddenly saw my daughter in my rearview mirror, sitting up, looking around, obviously aware of her surroundings. She immediately sank back into the little bed we had made in the rear of the station wagon, but I felt a tremendous sense of relief. She was alive, and she was in some kind of normal mental state!

My next anxiety was fear that I would make a mistake in finding my way to the hospital, but I didn't, and pulled up at the entrance to see my father, several attendants and a litter waiting for us.

It was clear after the first of these events that she was suffering from what I then thought of as epilepsy. I don't remember resisting this diagnosis or feeling any horror or shame over it. We were given rather an optimistic prognosis. The doctors told us that there was a good chance that this was a feature of adolescence and that she would grow out of it.

She got her license and drove a car at the normal age. So far as she and I can both remember, no one ever said anything about drinking—you don't to a thirteen-year-old—but her first non-nocturnal seizure came after an evening of partying at college. I remember having an acute discomfort at having to tell her she couldn't drive. She was driving us both somewhere just after a seizure, and I suddenly grasped the situation and felt compelled to tell her that she had to change places and let me drive. This is a tough message to give a teenager, and I remember that I did it awkwardly, probably causing more pain than necessary.

My daughter's illness has continued to be a major element in our lives. We have been fortunate in having time to be with her through extended hospital stays for testing and surgery. We are much more aware now of the relationship of her seizures to stress. We have also learned things about the human brain and its interaction with personality that have made us much more tolerant of human diversity.

50

Mother *Age 2½:* 10 days into measles (not German), my daughter became unconscious at 7 p.m. She was taken to the hospital, and in transport I noticed her eyes were wide open, pupils dilated, she had lost control of her bowels. The physician in the emergency room stated she had had a seizure. But, I commented, she did not twitch, not at all. She was taken to a medical center via ambulance, where she was examined, given blood tests and had a spinal tap. The pediatrician concluded she had measles encephalitis. The spinal tap was negative. She regained consciousness and was talking at about 10:30 p.m. She was given phenobarbital and a 50/50 chance to survive. After seven days of hospitalization, she was released. She was followed periodically thereafter—on no medication.

Age 6: Upon entering kindergarten a teacher recommended that we have a physician see my daughter and prescribe a drug for the difficulty she was having paying attention in class. She was on this drug until the age of puberty, approximately age 13–14, when she began to have migraine headaches. The medication was stopped.

Age 16: While attending school and occasionally at home my daughter felt like she was falling, also had a slight lightheadedness during a meeting. As a fainting spell, she did not lose consciousness.

Age 24: After marriage she began to show signs of stress, throwing her eyeglasses, banging her fists, and stating she was unaware she was doing this.   *1*

Living with Epilepsy

I was diagnosed with epilepsy after being told for over ten years that I didn't have it. It was very difficult for my parents to accept. And in some ways it was something that they did not want to really hear . . . because it made their daughter imperfect.

In the end, my mother blamed herself, because she had lifted a dresser while she was only eight-plus months pregnant with me. Because of that I was born premature.

Parents, DON'T BLAME YOURSELVES!!!!!!!!!!!!! It is not your fault that your child has epilepsy! And it is not the fault of brothers and sisters. Please, don't find fault with each other for something that you had nothing to do with. In the end, the person who feels the weight of all the guilt you try to lay on yourself or on the others in the family . . . is the one that has been diagnosed with epilepsy.

Just the other day, my mother admitted that she is still in a state of denial about my epilepsy. I was diagnosed over eight years ago!!!! How long can you deny something like this?! I was hurt when she told me. All this time she still has not accepted what happened to her "little girl." All I feel now is alone, and inadequate. I am no longer that "perfect child" that she gave birth to in her eyes. Having epilepsy is not easy for those of us with it. We tend to hide within ourselves what we feel about that word. It is like a label that we are given to wear for the rest of our lives, a label that many people do not like to hear . . . because they do not know what to say to us, or how to react to a seizure when it would occur.

For years, my seizures went undetected. I would always be tired when they were over, and I found that I could lay down for a few hours and be free from having another one. Sleep began to become an escape route for me . . . because in the end the seizures came every

Living with Epilepsy

hour . . . on the hour from the moment that I awoke in the morning. I used to long to be tired . . . just so that I could sleep and not have a seizure.

I have never forgotten what I went through. The hurt of losing friends because I acted strange at times. The anger that I would feel when I would be let go from a job . . . because I had seizures . . . but had been told by doctors that I was not having them. And the lonely feelings that I would get in the evenings, because no one would date the person with the problems.

I look back on what I went through with mixed emotions, some good, and some of them bad . . . but I look at what happened as a learning experience. Not so much for me, but for others. I would hate for someone to go through all of what I did.

I tell friends that if they see someone have a seizure . . . don't run away . . . like you did with me. Stay with the person, make sure that they do not get hurt in any way and *take notes*!!!!!!!!! Quite often someone with epilepsy does not know what they are doing when a seizure happens. If someone could just take notes of what they may see, or hear and tell the doctors it could mean a possible end to the recurrence of seizures in the future. And believe me, it will mean more to them than you could ever imagine. Don't be so afraid to help someone, by doing something so simple.

What is life like having seizures? I'm not able to drive and able to go places by myself. In a way I feel I have to depend on people too much to get around. Also I would like to do more things by myself. People think I'm in great pain during them from what I'm going through and the motions I'm making. One lady was on the verge of crying after she saw me have one. My father started talking to me and joking with me and I was just fine afterward.

You hear about IT as an aside to the lives of writers, artists and historical figures but no one knows how much epilepsy affected their lives . . . no one but the person with epilepsy.

The time has been long overdue for people to start listening to the challenge that having epilepsy creates. My personal case history with the disorder travels back to childhood. Tantrums and violent outbreaks with no memory recall gave the portrait of a "gifted child." The most traumatic developments hit rather late in my teens, then again in my late twenties and later to worsen in my mid to late thirties. I have always been an overachiever. When I am well (without having major convulsions) the world would seem to embrace my enthusiasm for life. When I fall into a seizure I may nearly die. Each time I emerge from "status epilepticus" there begins a reawakening to life.

I have waited so diligently for a neurologist who does not find me disdainful in their competitive practice to save and to cure.

I have seizures. I have been blessed to have worked with a neuropsychologist who knows me to be a vital struggling artist. I pray that I shall live long enough to see my plays performed and my poetry read by others.

I try to live my life in between seizures as normally as possible. I try very hard not to let having a seizure disorder affect my life at all. If I worried about having seizures, when I would have the next seizure, what would happen during it, etc., I would never leave my house. My attitude is "If it is going to happen, it's going to happen and until it does I do my best not to worry about it." I believe having

Living with Epilepsy

this attitude has enabled me to live independently for the past eight years.

I have found it best to let people I am in contact with (such as co-workers, support group members, etc.) know about my seizure disorder and what they should do if I have a seizure when I first come into contact with them, so if I should have a seizure, they are prepared and know how to handle it.

I am fortunate to have been employed full time for the past ten years. The company I work for was aware of my seizure disorder when I was hired, and there has never been any problem with my having a seizure disorder.

I think maintaining a good sense of humor has helped me a great deal in coping with my seizures over the past 27 years.

I feel very normal before I have one or a series of seizures. With my continuous seizures I get confused and repeat myself, sometimes I must stop what I am doing. When I have drop seizures I have no warning, cannot speak, just fall wherever I am, afterward I must orient myself before I can get up. Sometimes I feel frustrated and angry. I would like to live my life and be like any normal person, and be treated normally. It's like walking into a dark room and suddenly the light comes on. Sometimes I feel as though I am living in limbo, between heaven and hell.

To experience a seizure of any kind is an emotional and physical trauma. The fact that I must take daily medication to control my seizures reminds me of my illness. And, of course, those around me with their well meaning attitudes are forever reminding me of what I can't do because I have epilepsy. Not a day goes by when someone asks me if I'm taking my pills. I feel that I'm going to spend the rest of my life drugged—a prisoner of epilepsy. From a psychological point of view I view ladders, steps and other heights with the fear that I could experience a seizure and do harm to myself. Will an accident cause me to damage one of the many art works I have accumulated over a lifetime? Perhaps more than anything else I worry about having a seizure around friends. Though many people never mention it, I am aware that many regard my illness as frightening . . . too many people. Someone with epilepsy can never be a whole person.

Sometimes I get very frustrated and don't want to deal with the feeling of fear I get not knowing what I'm doing during a seizure and thinking in the back of my mind: what if I did this, what if I did that. I'm an emotional person (and it doesn't help if you're that type of person and you have a seizure disorder). The main thing is not to let it drag you down—talk to other people about it. I'm glad I know someone else who has epilepsy because when I find I'm having a hard time dealing with it I call her and she gets a lot of the same feelings I do. That helps me feel better and lets me know I'm not crazy. Sometimes I can either be overly friendly or overly upset.

I feel good about myself and could care less what other people think. A seizure is just a terrible interruption that I don't have control over. Most people are understanding about seizures, and the ones who aren't, well that's their problem.

Sometimes after a seizure I need to be reassured that I'm not losing it. I just hate that scary feeling that I get during some seizures. I just have to keep saying to myself—"Nobody can hurt you, just relax."

Living with Epilepsy

Life in between seizures. I am lucky for I have a husband who supports me and cares for me when I need it. However, I always feel that he and my family become worried and scared over little things—such as if I am not home on time or if I have been having trouble. This frustrates me because I know they may have reason to worry but I wish they didn't. I hate having others worry. I also feel incompetent when I can't get around and need to ask other people for a ride. Usually the people I ask are going my way, but I hate to ask. It is even worse if others have to accommodate me and go out of their way. This makes me feel like I am a pain in the ass to them.

The teasing and other statements that are said to me regarding my seizures make me feel less than human and more like a freak. A nurse where I work told me that I should wear a Big Black "X" across my chest to warn people to stay away from me because I may have a seizure around them. Others called me crazy Mary, yet others called me Scary Mary, all after watching me have a seizure. These became my nicknames whether I liked it or not. I would hear them down corridors at work or when I was in school. They made me feel inhuman.

I get very frustrated when I have a seizure after having gone a while without one. I feel like somehow it was my fault, even though I didn't do anything wrong.

My life between seizures is spent working 40 hours a week, sleeping a lot and being with my family. I find myself always feeling like I could nap. I know I have to sleep a while when I get home from work or I will be too tired to do anything else the rest of the night. If I don't get enough sleep, the next day at work I will be dragging. I generally will nap for 1 hour so my husband and I are able to spend time together and I feel fortunate that he is here, for he has accepted me when I'm tired, seizing or whatever. For that I feel lucky!

Having epilepsy gives me "mixed" feelings. On the one hand, I really hate being confined and limited since I had to stop driving a car 10 years ago at the age of 41. On the other hand, I've always been grateful my seizures are limited to "confusion spells" and "black-outs." I'm grateful I do not have convulsions. I am also grateful I was still able to drive a car when my children were younger and very involved in their school and church activities.

For reasons no one has been able to explain, medication has never completely controlled my seizures. I have several "confusion" spells daily, and have the "blackout" seizures approximately once a week.

I lead a normal life, but with limitations. I don't travel alone very often. I find not being able to drive a car anymore to be the most frustrating part to live with. I live where there is no public transportation available, so I am dependent on friends and acquaintances for rides. I am not within walking distance to a grocery store or my doctors. All my relatives live away, including my elderly mother who also lives alone and cannot drive long distances.

Because I can no longer drive, I do not feel in control of my life. I cannot go anywhere without calling someone for a ride. Some Sundays I have called five or six people before finding a ride to church. I get to a grocery store every four or five weeks. Weekly staples like bread or milk must be purchased at a convenient store where I must pay more for the items than I would in a grocery store.

I love to browse through stores and shop, and I rarely have the opportunity to do this. If I go out with someone else, we go where they want to go and leave when they choose to, not when I am ready.

My husband died eight years ago, and I am proud to say I am managing fairly well on my own. I am responsible for a three bedroom home with a large yard and gardens, and have had to learn how to maintain this on a limited income. It is not easy. When I feel sorry for the way I must live, I remind myself there are many others so much worse off and thank God I am able to function as well as I do.

The first time I ever found out I was having seizures was from a friend at work. I had just arrived home and my phone rang and she asked me if I was O.K. I asked her why and she told me that I was acting real strange in work today. So I went to the doctor. When the doctor first told me I was having seizures I could not believe it. I kept saying to myself this is a nightmare.

It was hard for me to adjust to this. I am glad that I have such a caring family and friends who have helped me to keep faith in this whole situation. For me to accept epilepsy is very hard. My whole life changed. My moods changed. I can't drive a car anymore. It's changed my whole personality. I hate looking to see the hurt it has put my family and my friends through. Sometimes I am afraid to go out in the public and have a seizure because it can be embarrassing.

I have had several seizures over the last year and a half. With each seizure, I would become more concerned, apprehensive and depressed. My parents have never witnessed any of my seizures, but I have told them what it felt like before and after experiencing the seizures. This condition has prevented me from obtaining employment, since most employment applications contain items asking about health and medications. This adds to my frustration and concern for the future.

I wouldn't say it's easy or fun to have epilepsy, because we never know when or where a seizure can occur, and this is very scary. Having to take several pills a day can be a drag. I get tired early and go to bed early and get up very early, so I'm on a weird schedule.

I work when work is available. Play softball, volleyball, bowl, and ride bikes. I went to school and graduated. I have friends and a good support system.

I guess the few problems I run into are tiredness and depression. And a few problems with people who are "ignorant about epilepsy." Most are understanding though, and I try to educate them.

Even so, I can function pretty well, thanks to the medication I'm on. In between seizures, my life is pretty normal like most people.

Living Safely with Epilepsy

Patricia Osborne Shafer, RN, MN

Nancy Santilli, BSN, MSN

Living safely with seizures can be challenging for many persons with epilepsy and their families. Safety and security are basic human needs, and when a person has a seizure, their safety and sometimes the safety of others may be threatened. Fortunately, as described in this chapter, there are many things that family members, friends, and co-workers can do to protect the person with epilepsy before and during a seizure and to comfort him or her afterwards. In addition, there are a number of things that the person with epilepsy can do. But even after being armed with safety information and putting it into practice, people may still have lingering fears or concerns about witnessing seizures or about the potential for injury occurring to a person during a seizure.

Epilepsy affects everyone who cares about or comes in contact with a person with seizures, as this book poignantly emphasizes. This chapter is structured around a few major safety concerns expressed by persons who have witnessed another person's seizures. Following each safety-related question are excerpts from contributors that highlight pertinent thoughts, concerns, and experiences. The authors then offer suggestions on how each problem may be managed. The chapter concludes with several lists of key safety pointers.

What should I do when a person has a seizure?

I was unable to move and was mesmerized by my son's expression; he no longer looked like a baby, but like a serious adult transfixed by the fear! 3b

I felt a wave of fear for him and scared because although I knew he had epilepsy, I wasn't sure what to do! (and I am a registered nurse!) 6

Witnessing a seizure, especially for the first time, can be very frightening and is likely to evoke feelings of helplessness or desperation. If the person having the seizure is someone you love or care for deeply, these feelings may be overwhelming. Unless you have been taught how to recognize what may occur during a seizure, you may not even be sure what is happening. For example, you may mistakenly think the person is having a heart attack or stroke.

Each person's reaction to witnessing a seizure will vary; however, staying calm is the most useful response for everyone. Hopefully after reading the rest of this chapter, you will know what to do during a person's seizure.

The first time I saw my teacher having a seizure I wasn't afraid or worried, because it was already explained to me. 9g

If people know what to expect, they are less likely to be afraid, can remain calm, and can give the appropriate assistance. Therefore, it is extremely important for persons with epilepsy to tell those with whom they have regular contact that they have seizures and what to do when one occurs. By sharing this information, the person with seizures will be able to move freely in the community with a greater sense of security, knowing that others are available to help. If a person's seizures are uncontrolled, it can be extremely helpful to alert local emergency teams (such as the rescue squad, fire department, police department, and emergency room staff) so they will be aware that the person is a member of the community and can note any special medical needs. This measure prevents unnecessary visits to the local emergency room.

There are two aspects to seizure first aid. The first is to provide "care and comfort" to the person having the seizure. This may involve giving physical assistance during the seizure and offering comfort and reassurance as the person recovers. Since each person's seizures are unique, the physical assistance that you can offer will be dictated by the behaviors the person shows during the seizure. The comfort measures that you should take will have to be explained to you by the person with epilepsy. The second part of seizure first aid for some people may involve intervening to help stop the seizure or help lessen its effects. This may not be possible in everyone. However, people who have an implanted device such as a vagus nerve stimulator may swipe a magnet over the implanted generator (usually located under the skin on the left side of the chest) which may shorten a seizure or lessen its severity. For people who are prone to clusters of seizures or long seizures, doctors may prescribe a medication that can be given in special circumstances. The goal of this type of intervention is to prevent seizures from becoming medical emergencies. They are not designed to take the place of emergency medical care when a true emergency is happening.

Assessing a person's safety during or after a seizure will depend on what kind of seizures they have. Since there are several types of seizures and not all seizures pose a risk of injury, it's often more appropriate to talk about seizure behaviors that affect safety rather than focus on specific seizure types. Seizure behavior falls into three general categories: staring episodes, physical manifestations with or without warning, and convulsions.

Staring Episodes

They complained that on several occasions when they spoke to her, she would ignore them. On one occasion I went up to their cubicle to pick up some work and one of them said, "I don't know what's wrong—but she is totally ignoring us." "When I went over to look at her, she was gazing into her computer screen. I called her name and she didn't respond . . . 40g

Staring episodes usually last only a few seconds to a minute. During that time the person is unaware of what is going on around him or her. It may be necessary to repeat directions or give assistance to protect the person from injury, such as preventing the person from standing still in the middle of a busy street instead of continuing to cross the street. These episodes usually go unnoticed unless they occur with such frequency that the person appears "spacey," "confused," and not quite "with it." In these circumstances, medical help may be needed to help stop prolonged events. Otherwise, just staying with the person until the staring stops and the person feels back to their normal self is usually all that is needed.

Physical Manifestations with or without Warning

When he has a seizure there is no warning. He just stops what he is doing. . . makes funny sounds and walks around. His right hand and arm seem to stiffen up and sometimes tremble, and sometimes he stares off into space and seems to lean to the right as if to fall, but he doesn't fall. He is in this position for about two to three minutes. Then he will wander around as if he is looking for something. After this, he takes off his clothes and looks for his pajamas and is still very incoherent and without a clue to where he is. After about five minutes of this he comes out of it and proceeds to do what he was doing before he had the seizure. 39

When he is going to have a seizure, he will say to me, "Uh, can you help me? I don't feel good"! 5b

It is important to respond according to the seizure behavior. If the person loses balance, assist him or her to a safe position, such as sitting in a chair or lying down on the floor. If the person begins walking or running, move objects out of the way to ensure a safe environment. If possible, keep them in an enclosed space so they don't wander into a dangerous situation. Talking calmly to the person during the seizure can be helpful in directing him to sit in a chair or stay in the room. In complex partial seizures, the person's awareness, ability to communicate, and recall may gradually recover and help the observer know when the seizure behavior is ending. If a person is fortunate enough to have a warning before a seizure, he can often position himself so as to avoid or minimize injury. Having a warning also gives him an opportunity to alert those around him that a seizure is beginning, or even intervene in certain situations, thus making the event less of a surprise.

Convulsions

I heard this whine, then a loud cry, and I said to myself that it must be my friend. I went over to see what was happening, and I saw that her face was red, she was shaking, her eyes were looking up at the ceiling, and she was pushing her mother away. Her mother was holding her. The whole time her face changed from red to a light gray/blue, and I freaked out. I felt like crying. I hadn't seen anyone in a long time have a seizure. I walked away because I felt so bad, since I couldn't do anything for her. 12a

A convulsion can be frightening to observe. The person's color may change and breathing stops momentarily or becomes very labored when chest muscles tighten. Time may seem to pass very slowly to an observer, when, in fact, it is going by more quickly. Helping the person to a safe position is vital. Catching him if he starts to fall down and supporting the head can minimize or prevent injury. Positioning the person to promote adequate breathing is critical and can be accomplished by turning the person on his side and positioning the head to keep an open airway. Body movements during a convulsion usually last no more than a couple minutes, yet the person may be difficult to arouse for several minutes or longer after the event. As he begins to return to his original physical state, the person may be disoriented for a short period of time and complain of a headache or muscle soreness.

It is not absolutely necessary to call an ambulance for assistance each time a person with epilepsy has a convulsion if that person is known by the observers to have had convulsions in the past. As a general rule, stay calm, don't panic, and stay with the person to make sure that he doesn't get hurt. Record the length of the seizure. Make mental notes of what you see or hear and give that information to the person having the seizure. Reassure onlookers that the person is just having a seizure and everything is under control. However, emergency help should be called if a seizure lasts five minutes or longer, if a second seizure occurs soon after the first one, or if the person was injured.

How else can I help someone during and after a seizure? I feel so useless.

She would want to be held closely until the seizure passed, a matter of a few minutes. 8b

Sometimes after a seizure I need to be reassured that I am not losing it. I just hate that scary feeling that I get during some seizures . . . and there are particular people (friends and families) that I have to talk to about it—mainly after a seizure.

Just asking a person with epilepsy what to do during and after a seizure will provide very useful information. Some persons may simply want someone to sit with them; others find it helpful to be talked to calmly. Still others may ask for a washcloth or tissue to wipe away any saliva that has come out of their mouths. Some persons may need to go to the bathroom after the seizure, so helping them to locate one can be very helpful. Others may want to lie down for a while.

When should I call an ambulance?

In certain situations, it is appropriate to call a rescue squad. Some people may have clusters of seizures that stop on their own. When this occurs in others, more than one seizure or long seizures may mean they are at risk for status epilepticus, a life-threatening situation. This is usually defined as a single convulsion lasting over 5 minutes or when the person has one seizure after another without regaining consciousness between episodes. Since treatment of status epilepticus requires emergency medical care, it is critical that family members, friends, and caregivers understand what to do in these situations. Ideally, people will have a plan in place that will alert others what to do if seizures look different than normal and who to call for help.

Emergency help may also be needed if any injury is suspected or observed, if a seizure occurs in water, or if the person requests it. If you come upon an unknown person who appears to be having a seizure, who is alone, and who does not have a Medic Alert bracelet or medical information on his person, you should offer care and comfort measures as previously described and call an ambulance to provide further assistance.

How can I tell if a person is okay after a seizure?

The actual end of the seizure is the most confusing part, in my opinion. In other words, it is sometimes hard to tell exactly when she is back on track. Many times I think she is functioning normally only to find out 10 to 20 minutes later that she doesn't recall anything that was said or done during that time period.   11d

After the seizure is over, he is generally anxious to assure us that he is fine, although it does seem that it takes him a few more minutes to completely regain his composure.   46c

Many people are unaware or unresponsive during or after a seizure. Determining when a person is safe to be alone or if extra help is needed can be difficult in these situations. Talking to a person during and after a seizure to reassure him that he is safe and to assess his level of awareness is essential to evaluating the need for support. Ask questions to determine if the person knows his and your name, where he is, what time of day it is, and what happened. If the person is not able to answer these questions, telling him this information may help decrease confusion and orient him to his surroundings. Before you leave the person alone, be sure that he is able to answer the who, what, when, and where questions.

Should I tell a person who has had a seizure what happened during the seizure?

After the seizure has passed, she has no memory of anything that has gone on, and oftentimes does not believe anything has happened.   2

I have seen this time after time with her. She tries so hard to be a normal person and hide the fact that she has epilepsy. She constantly denies the fact that she has had a seizure. It isn't until I take her step by step from beginning to end that she realizes that she really did have a seizure. I have gone over and over with her that it is vitally important for her to ask for help. 31a

Part of learning to live safely with seizures is knowing when to ask for help and telling others what is most helpful. If the person with seizures does not offer this information, family and friends should **ask** how they can best be of help. The sense of unpredictability and loss of control that a person with epilepsy may feel is often heightened by not knowing what occurs during a seizure. Some people may not want to talk about the seizures or may need time to gather their thoughts and feelings first. Others may feel scared, embarrassed, angry, or depressed after a seizure. These emotions can be part of the postictal phase or a consequence of feeling a loss of control. Nevertheless, when the person is ready, he should be told what happened during the seizure. However painful this may be, the information is helpful for the person and his health care providers to determine the type of seizures, effectiveness of treatment, and need for changes. Additionally, knowing what happened during a seizure and having a chance to talk about it may help make the seizures less scary and life seem more predictable.

Family members should not be surprised if the person expresses anger at the one who witnessed the seizure. I (POS) remember my own experiences as a child. I would always get angry at my mother. Why not? She was the one who saw the seizures, told me about them, and took me to the doctors. I couldn't see the seizures; thus I couldn't really get angry at them. I couldn't show my doctor how angry I was, either; I needed him to help me! So Mom was the target—the visible reminder of the seizures and the feeling that I was "different." Luckily she handled my anger fairly well. Her telling me about my seizures eventually helped me to understand them, adjust, and find a way to live safely with them. Life became more predictable and less scary as I knew what to expect. The information provided to me was invaluable as I "grew up" and assumed responsibility for my own health.

Should a child be permitted to see a parent have a seizure, and what should the child do?

I was 13 years old, on a visit to my grandparents, when I was told that my father had epilepsy, but I didn't know at that time what epilepsy was or what it had to do with me. When we got home, no one talked about what had been disclosed, and I couldn't seem to get the courage to bring it up. I was scared to be left alone with him, not knowing what a seizure was or what to do for someone experiencing one. All I knew was that I had to avoid him as much as possible so I wouldn't have to deal with the problem. 41c

Children can usually cope with witnessing seizures if they are properly taught what to do, just as they can be taught fire drills and other safety procedures. Although it is often easier for parents who have seizures to hide that fact from their children, it is usually better for the children if they are told about the seizures and even allowed to watch them. Children are likely to think that seizures are "bad" or scary if they are not allowed to witness one. They may fear that the parent is dying or abandoning them if the parent is hospitalized frequently because of seizures. Although these fears are understandable and sometimes unavoidable, they can be made more realistic and manageable if parents openly talk to their children about the seizures. This may help children realize that they are not alone in feeling scared, angry, or confused, and it is okay to ask questions and express their own feelings. In teaching children about seizures, parents may want to arrange for their children to view, either with the parents or a health care provider (or both), a videotape of seizures.

Families should be encouraged to hold "seizure drills"—a time to teach what seizures may look like, what to expect, and what to do should someone in the family have a seizure. Children can experience a full range of responses to their parent's seizures. Some children manage seizures well by themselves, whereas others may feel burdened with responsibility. Involving the child to help with age-appropriate responsibilities is usually best. A child as young as 3 years old can be taught to dial 911 or push a preprogrammed emergency number for help. Depending upon the circumstances, the family may choose a paging or emergency response system. Older children can be taught to hold a parent's hand, offer reassurance, or provide more direct safety assistance.

It is also helpful for children to meet the parent's health care providers. A child may ask a doctor, nurse, or social worker questions that he would not ask the parents. Health care providers may have age-appropriate materials to teach children about seizures and first aid. The Epilepsy Foundation (www.epilepsyfoundation.org or 800-332-1000) and *epilepsy.com* (www.epilepsy.com) also has many materials for families and children of all ages.

Can a person with seizures be allowed to drive a car?

The main concern about driving and seizures is, and should be, safety—for the driver with seizures, passengers, and the general public. Another concern is freedom—a driver's license confers freedom and independence. Not being able or permitted to drive can adversely affect many aspects of a person's life—work, finances, family and parenting, socialization, and emotional well-being.

Each state has its own laws regulating the licensing of drivers. The laws pertaining to seizures and driving vary from state to state with most requiring a person to be seizure-free for a period of three months to one year before being issued a driver's license. In some places, health care providers must report every person with seizures whereas in other states self-reporting is the rule.

Persons with epilepsy should talk to their doctor about their seizures and ability to drive, and be aware of the licensing requirements in their state, province, or country. People who do not follow these regulations may be assuming significant legal, safety, and financial risks. If a person with seizures and his doctor's perceptions of the person's ability to drive disagree with state regulations, the person may contact the Medical Advisory Board of his state's Department of Motor Vehicles. Further information about driving and epilepsy may be obtained from local epilepsy organizations, the Epilepsy Foundation, and transportation departments.

How can I help a person live safely with seizures?

For my son there were many crashes to the floor or in the shower. There were police incidents; work-related accidents; calls from the school to have him brought home; loss of jobs; driver's license, friends. 14a

He has always had a lot of freedom; he has taken public transportation by himself since he was 6 years old, and I let him do all kinds of sports, in which he succeeds extremely well. Also, my son maintains his self-confidence and is very optimistic. 3b

We all take risks when we get into a car, ride a bike, walk to school, or cross a street. Risks are a part of life. People with epilepsy and their families must accept risks just like everyone else. However, they may also be faced with accepting the risk of injury from a seizure and the risks of side effects of medicines or other treatments. Before families can accept these risks, they must work with their health care providers to talk about their fears and realistically assess actual or potential risks to their safety. A safety management plan can then be developed with strategies to decrease the potential for injury. This may help people put risks and safety issues into proper perspective and enable people with epilepsy and their families to feel more in control of their lives.

Various types of injuries and accidents may occur from seizures, such as cuts or lacerations, fractures, sprains, bruises, and burns. Choking can occur if the person has a seizure while eating. Also, inappropriate first aid for a seizure may result in airway obstruction and choking. Even more serious is the potential for drowning. People can drown in as little as a few inches of water. We don't like to think about these more serious kinds of injuries and accidents, but we must if we want to think about ways to decrease the chances of their happening.

Living safely with seizures may entail modifications in the lifestyle, environment, or both of the person with epilepsy—changes designed to prevent injury, minimize triggers of seizures, increase predictability of seizures, and enhance independence in daily life. The first step in safety management is to assess the risk of injury in relation to the seizure behaviors, frequency of seizures, the type of activities the person wants to pursue, and the skills required to perform those activities. Other areas that should be considered include predictability, opportunities to minimize or prevent injury, and the person's willingness to use recommended safety measures. Once these factors have been evaluated, families can implement appropriate safety management measures.

There are many simple and practical safety measures that people can take to prevent injury and remain independent. For example, kitchens and bathrooms are often sites of injury. People can burn their hands on a stove during a seizure or under running hot water. Burns from stoves can be prevented by wearing long-handed mitts while cooking, using back burners, and using burner covers when the stove is not in use. Burns from running hot water can be decreased by re-setting the thermostat to prevent scalding and having an automatic water shut-off installed. Additional safety tips are given at the end of this chapter. Safety management ideas are limited only by one's imagination.

Living safely with seizures is a challenge—one that is not talked about enough. First aid for seizures should focus on the seizure behaviors that affect safety. In this chapter, examples of staring episodes (absence seizures), physical manifestations with or without warning (complex partial seizures), and convulsions (generalized tonic-clonic seizures) were discussed. Caring for a person during a seizure may involve providing physical assistance and comfort measures individualized to the person's seizure behaviors and desires. Ways to intervene and stop seizures early or lessen their severity may be possible for some people. Living safely with seizures will also depend on people with epilepsy and their families having a "take charge" approach to assess and manage their lifestyle and environment in the safest way possible. By so doing, persons with epilepsy and their families can continue to live full, active, and relatively independent lives.

Safety Tips for Persons with Epilepsy

Bathing Tips

- Use nonskid strips in tub or shower.
- Use tub or shower chair, or sit on bottom of tub and use handheld shower nozzle.
- Use tub rails or grab bars.
- Avoid baths—fill tub no higher than the length of your nose!
- Check that drain works properly in shower.
- Never take a shower or bath alone (have someone in the house if possible). *Regularly singing* in the shower helps alert another person that you are safe.

- Keep hot water temperature low to avoid burns, and always check water temperature before entering shower. If sensation is poor, have someone else check it.
- Use padded covers on heaters to avoid burns.
- Use an electric razor to avoid cuts.
- Use plastic bottles and containers to avoid cuts from broken glass.
- Hang bathroom door so it opens out—this will allow people to easily get in to help.

Dressing Tips

- Avoid accessories with sharp edges.
- Store clothes at an easy-to-reach height to avoid climbing.
- If you have difficulty with attention, sorting, organizing, or other visual-spatial skills, keep clothes organized by type of outfit, color, or season.

Eating Tips

- Make sure that caregivers, friends, or family know how to assist someone who is choking.
- Always eat sitting upright. Use chairs with armrests to prevent falls.
- Use nonskid surfaces under plates and cups to avoid spills.
- Use a bowl or scoop dish if coordination is a problem.
- Use a cup with a lid and spout (i.e., commuter cup) for warm liquids.
- Use nonbreakable dishes.

Safety in the Home

- Keep hallways and rooms free from clutter.
- Avoid sharp corners or use padding on corners and edges of furniture.

- Use thick padding under carpets. Use wall-to-wall carpeting on all floors. Avoid throw rugs.
- Avoid ironing or iron only if someone else is present; an iron with automatic shut-off is recommended.
- Keep sharp utensils in safe places to avoid cuts.
- Remove burner controls on stove except when cooking or avoid controls that could be turned on easily by accident.
- Use microwave oven and microwaveable cookware and dishes whenever possible.
- Use long oven mitts and back stove burners in order to avoid burns resulting from knocking something off front burners.
- Keep all toxic cleaning agents out of kitchen and bathroom, preferably in *locked* cabinets.
- Use rubber gloves to wash dishes.
- Store frequently used items at a convenient height. Avoid climbing.
- Use a cart to transport dishes and hot foods.
- Use a vegetable chopper or food processor to avoid cutting with a knife, or buy precut frozen or canned foods.
- Use a colander basket with handles to lift cooked foods out of hot water; let water cool before moving pan.
- Limit number of pillows if person has tendency to seizures during sleep.
- Consider using a monitor or alarm to alert family members to seizures at night.
- Lock doors for people who tend to wander during seizures.

Recreation Tips

- Use *common sense* in recreation; avoid rock climbing, parachuting, skydiving, scuba diving, hang gliding, and unsupervised swimming or skiing.

Living Safely with Epilepsy

- Make sure that friends and family know epilepsy first aid.
- Always have a "buddy" for activities that require considerable exertion or that are likely to cause injury.
- Take frequent breaks and drink plenty of water.
- Wear protective clothing (elbow or knee pads, protective eyeglasses or goggles) whenever possible.
- When bike riding, avoid busy streets; ride on bike paths or side streets, always wear a helmet, and ride with a partner. *Don't* ride if you have frequent seizures or if your coordination is poor.
- Use a helmet for any contact sport, bike riding, or other activities when needed.
- When swimming or boating, always wear a life jacket. Swim with a friend and only if your doctor approves.
- Play on soft surfaces (grass, mats, carpets) whenever possible.
- Avoid open flames. Sit far back from campfires and stoves and be in the company of others who know what to do if you have a seizure.
- Exercise in a cool room or, if outdoors, in the early morning or evening, to avoid the hottest part of the day.
- Avoid small, overcrowded spaces that are not well ventilated or free from objects.
- Use seat belts in cars and do not drive unless you have your doctor's permission and meet the legal criteria for your state.
- ALWAYS CARRY A MEDIC ALERT CARD, BRACELET OR NECKLACE.
- Consider computerized emergency medical information.

When Parent Has Seizures

- Child-proof house—get down on the floor to assess safety risks to parent and children.

- Avoid sleep deprivation; have spouse help with night-time feedings.
- Take naps when child naps; ask family or friends for help.
- Never bathe child alone.
- Place baby on carpeted floor to change diapers or clothes.
- Use stroller to transport infant or small child, rather than carrying child.
- Use a backpack baby carrier only if you do not have falling seizures.
- Use disposable diapers, to avoid safety pins.
- Keep diapers, toys, and playpen on each floor of home, to avoid unnecessary stair climbing.
- KEEP ALL MEDICATIONS IN CHILDPROOF BOTTLES AND OUT OF REACH OF CHLDREN.

Further Reading

1. Clerico C. Occupational therapy and epilepsy. *Occupational therapy in health care.* 1989;6:41–74.

2. Golden R et al. *Safe Living with Seizure Disorders—Ideas for the Home.* Comprehensive Epilepsy Program, Health Sciences Center, University of Virginia, Charlottesville, Virginia. 1986.

Index

attitude, positive, 83, 99–100, 101

auras, 2, 61, 62, 63, 69

awareness

    evaluation of, and patient
        assistance, 112

    lack of, during seizures, 2, 8, 19,
        41, 93

    postictal period and, 3

    during seizures, 46, 55

balance issues, 12, 20, 54, 86, 109.
    See also falling down

bathing, and safety, 119, 122

bathroom visits, 38, 48, 111. *See also*
    bowel incontinence; urination

behaviors, seizure-related

    misdiagnoses of, 14, 45, 72, 93

    misinterpretations of, 28, 35, 38,
        67–68

    patient excuses for, 17, 55

    unusual postictal, 15, 39, 67

blackouts, 18, 48, 62, 63, 103

blanking out, 17, 18, 23, 25, 36, 38,
    40, 41, 49, 54, 55, 58, 62, 64,
    66, 89

blinking, of eyes, 24, 28, 32, 62

blueness, of lips, 50, 51

body issues. *See also* buckling, of legs;
    falling down; feet rocking;
    finger movements; fist
    clenching; furrowing, of
    eyebrows; hand motions;
    shaking; twitching

    jerking, 45, 49, 52, 59, 80

    limpness, 63

    one side reactions, 21–25, 63, 67,
        81, 87, 91

    rigidity, 8, 11, 15, 21, 42, 88

    temperature, 9, 37, 38

thumbs rubbing against index
    fingers, 27

unsteadiness, 11

urination, 12, 39, 54, 62

bowel incontinence, 54, 93

boyfriends, as seizure witnesses, 49

brain

    issues/involvement of, 1, 2, 3, 14,
        28, 66, 77

    surgery on, 61–62, 73, 77, 80, 92

breathing issues, 9, 50, 51, 59,
    63, 110

brothers

    as patients, 20–21

    as seizure witnesses, 41

buckling, of legs, 16, 58, 59

burns

    of hands, 18, 43, 118

    prevention of, 118, 119, 120

case managers, as seizure witnesses,
    87–88

chewing motion, 18, 19, 27, 29, 30,
    48, 67

children

    with brothers as patients, 20–21

    education and emergency
        instructions for, 115

    with fathers as patients, 21, 74–75,
        75–79

    infants as patients, 9, 31, 32,
        44, 89

    with mothers as patients,
        19–20, 65

    responsibility role reversals of,
        74–75, 78

    safety measures and, 122

    as seizure witnesses, 16–17, 35,
        114–115

choking, 13, 46, 117, 119
clothing
    organization of, 119
    for protection, 121
    removal of, 67, 109
clusters (multiple seizures)
    descriptions of, 11, 33, 42–43, 48,
        68, 79, 86, 88
    emergency assistance and, 111
cognitive processes. *See also*
        awareness; memory issues;
        verbal communication of
        patients
    activity continuation, during
        seizure, 37–38
    activity continuation, postictal, 24,
        61, 67
    brain fog, 48, 54
    impairments during seizure, 56,
        58, 66
    postictal impairments, 9, 67, 83
comfort measures, 107
communication. *See also* verbal
        communication of patients
    children and, 75–76, 114–115
    patient disclosures to associates,
        56, 83, 100, 107
    seizure details to patient,
        113–114
complex partial seizures (physical
        manifestations), 2–3, 109, 118
concentration, 56, 58
confinement, 103
confusion. *See also* disorientation
    daily, 103
    as indication of mild seizure, 56
    postictal, 37, 38, 43, 51
    during seizure, 69, 70, 100
    as seizure warning, 89

consciousness, loss of, 2, 16, 19, 54,
        66, 93
convulsions. *See also* grand mal
        seizures; secondarily
        generalized seizures; shaking;
        tonic-clonic seizures
    as beginning phase, 2
    danger of, 111
    descriptions of, 16, 32, 63,
        80–81, 81
    duration of, 16, 81
    recovery from, 3
    and safety, 110–111
    as secondarily generalized
        seizure, 2
convulsions, febrile, 32
cooking, and safety, 120
coping
    by children, 114
    by family members, 71
    by patient, 100
coughing, 12, 53
co-workers, 17, 29, 64–65,
        67–68, 104
crying
    by child, 31
    by family members, 76
    by friend, 31
    by husband, 16
    at seizure observation, 110
    during seizures, 82–83, 90, 110

daughters
    as patients, 8, 10–11, 18–19,
        27–28, 37–38, 40, 45–46,
        49–50, 52–53, 55, 58, 61–62,
        81–82, 86–87, 89, 91–93, 97
    as seizure witnesses, 65, 74–75,
        75–79, 80

clutching of, 59
dilation of, 30, 79
fixation/motionlessness of, 61, 81, 87
glassiness of, 15, 38, 70
glazing over of, 12, 13, 43
looking up/to side, 31, 47, 81, 110
rolling of, 21, 50, 89
spasms of eyelids, 9
turning of, 9, 47, 88, 89
twitching of, 62, 63
unfocusing of, 86
wide openness of, 58, 60, 93

face/facial expressions
blankness, 38, 40, 49, 62
confusion, 36
contortion, 42
dumbfounded, 19
faraway looks, 40
grinning/smiling, 39, 48
muscle tension, 41
sadness, 82
softness/relaxation, 66
spasms/twitching, 9, 11
subdued/somber, 55
withdrawn, 60
facial coloring, changes to
to blue to black, 59
during convulsions, 110
pale, 15, 40, 63, 87, 88
to red, 59, 84, 110
from red to blue, 31, 110
falling down. *See also* buckling, of legs
backwards, 54
drop seizures, 16, 90, 100
general, 34, 35, 42, 50, 57, 83, 84–85, 87, 89
injuries during, 46, 54, 72, 90

as seizure trigger, 11
from sitting position, 50, 88
from standing position, 33, 55
fathers
as patients, 21, 62, 74–75, 75–79
as seizure witnesses, 44–45, 54, 88–89, 90
fatigue
general, 102, 105
postictal, 19–20, 26, 33, 54, 63, 64, 80, 81
as seizure warning, 69
fear
of boyfriend, 49
of children, 21, 76, 80, 115
of family, 102
of in-laws, 70–71
of mothers, 43, 50, 59, 87, 90
of patients, 3, 18, 46, 51, 70, 76, 101, 113
of siblings, 20
of spouses, 16, 18, 81
of strangers, 32
of students, 22, 24, 25, 26
feet rocking, 27
fever, as seizure trigger, 1, 16, 32
fiancés, as seizure witnesses, 66
finger movements, 27, 29
first aid for seizures, 107
fist clenching, 27, 29
foaming at mouth, 12, 21, 41, 42, 54
fog, brain, 48, 54
forgetfulness, 7–8
freedom, lack of, 103
frequency of seizures, 8, 15, 22, 33, 38, 68
friends
appreciation of, 104
dependency on, 103

friends (*continued*)
    as limitation reminders, 100–101
    loss of, 35, 98
    seizure information
        communication to, 56, 83,
            100, 107, 111–112, 113, 121
    as seizure witnesses, 8–9, 29–31,
        37, 50–52, 54–57, 60,
        82–86
    social life sacrifices, 72, 78
    as support, 105
frustration
    of patients, 39, 100, 101, 102, 104
    of relatives, 12, 35, 36, 53, 82
furrowing, of eyebrows, 19

gagging, 44
gasping, 32
giggling, 84
God, faith in, 35
goose-bumps, 37
grabbing objects, 62
grand mal seizures, 44
gratitude, 60, 61, 70, 103
grinning, 39
groaning, 15
grocery shopping, 103
guilt, 35, 47, 85, 97
gulping, 8

hand motions
    claw-like, 50
    fist clenching, 27, 29
    movement of, 58
    pushing away objects, 86
    rubbing together, 39
    stiffening, 62, 67
    tremors/shaking, 34, 40, 54, 56,
        67, 87

head
    dropping, 88
    "funny feelings" in, 73
    moving around, 58
    turning to side, 22–26, 42, 88
    twitching, 55
headaches
    after convulsions, 110
    postictal, 14, 17, 21, 36, 38, 52,
        80, 81
    as seizure warnings, 37, 44, 48
head injuries, as seizure triggers,
    43, 46
hearing, 8, 19, 46, 88
held, desire to be, 18
helplessness
    of husbands, 18, 69
    of mothers, 35, 61, 90
    of patients, 56
    of siblings, 20, 21, 53
    of students, 24
heroism, 85
"Holy Man disease," 71
humor, 19, 100
husbands
    as patients, 13–15, 16–17, 21,
        38–39, 47–49, 64, 72–74,
        79–80
    as seizure witnesses, 7–8, 18,
        56–57, 62–64, 68–70
hyperactivity, 37, 44

illnesses
    postictal nausea, 17, 40
    as seizure trigger, 1, 10, 16, 45
    as seizure warnings, 12, 13, 15
independence
    creation/maintenance of, 75, 78,
        99–100, 118

mothers
  as patients, 19–20, 65
  as seizure witnesses
    of daughters, 8, 10–11, 18–19,
      27–28, 37–38, 40, 45–46,
      49–50, 52–53, 55, 58, 61–62,
      81–82, 86–87, 89, 91–93, 97
    of infants, 9–10
    of sons, 11–13, 17, 26–27,
      32–35, 41–42, 43–44
mothers-in-law, as seizure witnesses,
  70–71, 71
motionlessness, during seizure, 61
mouth issues
  dryness, 58
  foaming, 12, 21, 41, 42, 54
  placing objects in, 46
multiple seizures. See clusters
  (multiple seizures)
muscle soreness/stiffness, 81, 88,
  89, 110
music, as seizure trigger, 1

nausea/vomiting, 14, 17, 40, 88, 91
nephews, as seizure witnesses, 87
note taking, of seizures/symptoms,
  91, 98, 110

optimism, 10

patients. See also daughters; sons
  acceptance by, 10, 46, 104
  advice from, 98
  anger of, 98, 100, 114
  brothers as, 20–21
  communication to others, 100, 101
  cousins as, 36
  daughters as, 8, 10–11, 18–19,
    27–28, 37–38, 40, 45–46,

      49–50, 52–53, 55, 58, 61–62,
      81–82, 86–87, 89, 91–93
  denial by, 17, 35, 55, 56, 64
  embarrassment of, 3, 52–53, 104
  fathers as, 21, 62, 74–75, 75–79
  fear of, 3, 18, 46, 51, 70, 76,
    101, 113
  guilt of, 97
  helplessness of, 56
  husbands as, 13–15, 16–17, 21,
    38–39, 47–49, 64, 72–74,
    79–80
  independence of, 10, 100, 103
  infants as, 9, 31, 32, 44, 89
  lack of social life, 98
  lifestyle normalcy, 99–100, 105
  limitations of, 98, 103
  mothers as, 19–20, 65
  positive attitudes of, 99–100,
    101
  public seizures of, 3, 18, 52–53, 83,
    101, 104
  as role models, 85
  screaming by, 33, 44, 75–76
  seizure descriptions, 99, 100
  worrying by, 101, 102
personality changes, 17, 56, 104
perspiration, 10, 13, 27, 42, 88, 89
petit mal seizures, 53
physical manifestations (complex
    partial seizures), 2, 109, 118.
    See also specific types of physical
    manifestations
physicians. See doctors
playing with objects, 62
positive attitude, 83, 99–100, 101
postictal periods (recovery)
  activity continuation, 24, 61, 67
  apologizing, 84

Index

Index

135

CPSIA information can be obtained at www.ICGtesting.com
Printed in the USA
LVOW10s1925310314

379680LV00009B/822/P